EMERGENCY CAPNOGRAPHY

This portable and practical pocket guide explains how capnography works both physiologically and electronically and helps clinical staff to apply the tool promptly and correctly, and to interpret appropriately the numeric and graphic displays, providing vital information when viewed in the context of the patient's clinical presentation, history, and other diagnostic data that will improve and enhance care.

Initial chapters explain how to interpret the data displayed in the context of various conditions, and how the care provider may respond to that data. Later chapters provide partial differential diagnoses based on the displayed capnometry data, an algorithm for interpreting waveforms, and clinical scenarios to illustrate the application of capnography in emergency medical practice.

Ensuring that the value of capnography can be maximized to the benefit of patients, the book is an essential primer to capnography for those studying for and practicing within the emergency medical services, and a convenient reference for other emergency department personnel.

EMERGENCY CAPNOGRAPHY

Hugh Greenbaum, BS, NRP

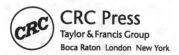

CRC Press
Taylor & Francis Group
Boca Raton London New York

CRC Press is an imprint of the
Taylor & Francis Group, an **informa** business

First edition published 2025
by CRC Press
2385 NW Executive Center Drive, Suite 320, Boca Raton FL 33431

and by CRC Press
4 Park Square, Milton Park, Abingdon, Oxon, OX14 4RN

CRC Press is an imprint of Taylor & Francis Group, LLC

ISBN: 978-1-032-79347-4 (hbk)
ISBN: 978-1-032-79346-7 (pbk)
ISBN: 978-1-003-49157-6 (ebk)

DOI: 10.1201/9781003491576

Typeset in Bembo Std
by KnowledgeWorks Global Ltd.

To Dr. Arthur Bernstein, MD
Cardiologist, Grandpa

Louis Allen Greenbaum
Engineer, Dad

Thank you for your inspiration!

CONTENTS

PREFACE

MOTIVATION

This book is written primarily for Emergency Medical Services (EMS) and emergency department personnel to help them make better decisions about patient care in the critical early minutes of patient encounters. My goals of writing this book are to

- Educate emergency medical providers at all levels in the capabilities and limitations of capnography.
- Make it easier for providers to understand what their capnography device, in conjunction with the patient's other signs and symptoms, is telling them, and to make the best use of the data.

This book is intended to fill in the gap between the very basic information about capnography that is found in EMS, nursing, and medical textbooks and the very detailed information that is found in medical journals and specialist textbooks. The basic version leaves providers without enough information to make the most of capnography, and the medical journals and specialist texts are hard to find, often expensive, and difficult to distill down to the guidance providers need.

CAVEATS

Capnography is a tool, not "The" tool. It provides good data for the provider regarding the patient's status, but the data must be used in conjunction with data from other devices (e.g., vital sign monitors, electrocardiography), and from the patients themselves (e.g., symptoms, medical, and medication history) along with the provider's medical judgment to make informed patient care decisions.

Specific treatments are mentioned as recommendations. Nothing in this text authorizes providers to deviate from their local protocols or scope of practice.

Specific brands are mentioned in the text. These provide examples and are not intended to be (nor should they be interpreted as) endorsements.

Opinions expressed herein are strictly mine and may not reflect the views of organizations or people with whom I am affiliated.

I have no conflicts of interest to disclose.

Hugh Greenbaum, BS, NRP

ACKNOWLEDGMENTS

Thank you to the staff at the Chesterfield County Fire and EMS Department Training Division, Chesterfield County, Virginia, especially Captain Jason Coleman, Amanda Danahy, and Qadira Stewart for their support.

I thank the following people who provided comments on drafts of this book. Any problems you find herein are strictly mine.

- Alice Beachy, MEd, EMT-Intermediate
- Terry Brooks, CRNA
- Captain Darren De Fluiter, MA, Firefighter/Paramedic
- Francis J. Diskin, MD
- Eric Edwards, MD
- Anthony Marant III, BA, NRP
- Martha Murphy, BS
- Rachel Toombs, MS, EMT
- Gail Weatherford, NP, NRP

AUTHOR

Hugh Greenbaum is an Emergency Medical Services (EMS) paramedic with Forest View Volunteer Rescue Squad, a 9-1-1 response agency in the US State of Virginia, with more than 39 years of experience as a volunteer EMS provider. He is certified as an EMS Education Coordinator in Virginia and teaches Emergency Medical Technician (EMT) classes for his agency. He holds a Bachelor of Science degree in Information and Computer Science from the University of California, Irvine. He was a part-time faculty member in the Department of Computer Science at California State University, Fullerton, and retired from a 40-year career in systems and software engineering.

ACRONYMS AND ABBREVIATIONS

°C	Degrees Celsius
°F	Degrees Fahrenheit
AHA	American Heart Association
ATP	Adenosine Triphosphate
BA	Bachelor of Arts
BS	Bachelor of Sciences
Ca^{+2}	Calcium Ions
cm H_2O	Centimeters of Water
CNS	Central Nervous System
CO_2	Carbon Dioxide
COPD	Chronic Obstructive Pulmonary Disease
CPR	Cardio-Pulmonary Resuscitation
CRNA	Certified Nurse Anesthetist
DKA	Diabetic Ketoacidosis
DOPE	Dislodgement, Obstruction, Placement, Equipment
EKG	Electrokardiogram
EMS	Emergency Medical Services
EMT	Emergency Medical Technician
$ETCO_2$	End-Tidal Carbon Dioxide
H^+	Hydrogen ion (i.e., a proton)
H_2CO_3	Carbonic Acid
H_2O	Water
HCO_3	Bicarbonate
I:E	Inspiratory–Expiratory Ratio

kPa	Kilopascals
LVAD	Left Ventricular Assist Device
MA	Master of Arts
MAP	Mean Arterial Pressure
MDMA	3,4–Methylenedioxymethamphetamine
MEd	Master of Education
mg/dL	Milligrams per deciliter
mL	Milliliters
mm	Millimeters
mmHg	Millimeters of Mercury
$NaHCO_3$	Sodium Bicarbonate
NIH	National Institutes of Health (United States)
NP	Nurse Practitioner
NRP	National Registry Paramedic (United States)
O_2	Oxygen
$PaCO_2$	Partial pressure of carbon dioxide dissolved in blood
PaO_2	Partial pressure of oxygen dissolved in blood
PCP	Phencyclidine
PEEP	Positive End-Expiratory Pressure
pH	Measure of hydrogen ions in blood
ROSC	Return of Spontaneous Circulation
RSI	Rapid Sequence Intubation
RVAD	Right Ventricular Assist Device
SpO_2	Peripheral oxygen saturation; Percentage of bound hemoglobin
V/Q	Ventilation versus Perfusion
VAD	Ventricular Assist Device
UTI	Urinary Tract Infection

BASIC CAPNOGRAPHY REVIEW

This chapter discusses what capnography is, the need for capnography, the associated anatomy and physiology, how capnography works, and how to use it.

1.1 WHAT IS CAPNOGRAPHY?

Capnography is a system that continuously measures exhaled carbon dioxide (CO_2). This measurement provides a real-time indication of the patient's ventilation, perfusion, and metabolism. Cyclic changes in the CO_2 flow are monitored to yield breaths per minute, the patient's ventilatory rate. Changes in the amount of exhaled CO_2 may indicate disturbances in ventilation, perfusion, and/or metabolism. The amount of exhaled CO_2 is displayed graphically (a capnogram), which allows for monitoring with each breath and trends over time. The amount of CO_2 measured at the end of each breath (end-tidal CO_2 [$ETCO_2$]) provides an indication of the patient's immediate perfusion and metabolic status (Ward & Yealy, 1998).

1.2 WHY DO WE NEED CAPNOGRAPHY?

There are three vital bodily functions that providers need to evaluate to understand a patient's condition and therefore how best to treat the patient: Ventilatory status, perfusion,

DOI: 10.1201/9781003491576-1

and metabolism. These functions are difficult to evaluate in the field and may require time-consuming laboratory work to evaluate in the emergency department.

The patient's *ventilatory status* can be difficult to evaluate with just eyes and ears. The patient's body habitus can make it difficult to hear lung sounds with even amplified stethoscopes. Lung sounds may be difficult to hear or evaluate due to lack of air flow; i.e., the patient does not breathe deeply enough to create enough turbulence for us to hear the characteristics of the flow. The patient's ventilatory rate can be difficult to evaluate visually due to clothing or blankets, bouncing in the back of the ambulance, the patient changing their breathing when they know they are being watched, or lack of visual clues (e.g., unlabored but shallow ventilation). Pulse oximetry can show the patient's oxygen saturation (SpO_2) is low, but not why. It can take more than one minute for fingertip pulse oximeters to indicate a dangerous drop in circulating oxygen (O_2) levels due to decrease in ventilation (including apnea) (Choi et al., 2010).

Tools are available to measure oxygen and glucose in the bloodstream, but they do not measure how well these are being distributed to the vital organs. Neither do they measure how well waste products, in particular CO_2 and metabolic acids, are being removed. In other words, they do not measure *perfusion*. Lack of perfusion to the organs (hypoperfusion) is the definition of the life-threatening condition known as shock (Ward, 2011). Tachycardia and hypotension are often used as surrogates for hypoperfusion. Many conditions other than shock can cause tachycardia, and hypotension is a late sign of shock (NAEMT & ACS, 2019).

The third vital function is how well oxygen and glucose are being used by the organs and how well waste products are being gathered and excreted, i.e., the body's *metabolism*. The human body operates in relatively narrow acid–base balance. Metabolic disturbances can upset this delicate balance. These conditions need to be identified and quickly corrected.

These vital functions can be evaluated by capnography. To understand how it works, it is necessary to review the anatomy and physiology of ventilation, perfusion, and metabolism.

1.3 ANATOMY AND PHYSIOLOGY REVIEW

All human organ systems rely on a steady supply of oxygen (O_2) and glucose in order to function properly. Oxygen is brought into the body via the respiratory system and glucose via the digestive system. Oxygen and nutrients are transported to the organs via the bloodstream. The cells within the organ systems metabolize these nutrients into various waste products, including CO_2, water (H_2O), and acids, which are carried away for disposal via the bloodstream. The following sections describe the anatomy and physiology of ventilation, perfusion, and metabolism, and tie them together to provide the basis for understanding the utility and limitations of capnography.

1.3.1 Ventilation

When the entire respiratory system (central nervous system, airway, lungs, and associated musculature) is working properly, the body can *ventilate*, that is bring air and its constituent O_2 into the body (inhale) and push waste gases out of the body (exhale). Various disease and traumatic processes can compromise the body's ability to ventilate; some of these are described in later chapters. The provider's challenge is to recognize that ventilation has been compromised, the type of compromise, the degree of compromise, and potential mechanisms for the compromise.

1.3.2 Perfusion

For the organs to function properly, they must be supplied, that is *perfused*, with a steady supply of oxygenated blood with available glucose. This same blood supply must be able to carry the waste products away from the cells for excretion. Perfusion depends on having an intact central nervous system and circulatory system, sufficient blood pressure to ensure blood reaches all of the organs, sufficient number of intact red blood cells to carry O_2 and waste gases, and an intact and properly functioning heart.

1.3.3 Metabolism

For organs to function, their individual cells must properly utilize, i.e., metabolize O_2 and nutrients, in particular glucose, to create the energy to perform their requisite functions. This process is known as the Krebs Cycle. When cells have sufficient oxygen, they perform aerobic metabolism to convert O_2 and glucose to adenosine triphosphate (ATP), with CO_2, water, and heat as waste products.

When cells are not properly perfused, they switch to anaerobic metabolism, where glucose and fats are metabolized into ATP, with lactic acid, water, and heat as waste products. The lack of proper blood flow means that both CO_2 from adequately perfused cells and lactic acid from inadequately perfused cells build up in the organs, which can lead to their failure and eventual death.

Various conditions can lead to adequately perfused cells improperly using the available nutrients, which lead to metabolic disturbances. These disturbances often manifest as acid–base imbalances. A classic example of a metabolic acid–base disturbance is diabetes mellitus, where the cells cannot ingest glucose. This leads to the cells using O_2 and fats to create ATP, with acidic ketones, H_2O, and heat as waste products. Left untreated, this leads to diabetic ketoacidosis.

1.3.4 Where ventilation, perfusion, and metabolism meet

When the body is in homeostasis, O_2 is carried to the cells and CO_2 is carried away by hemoglobin in the red blood cells. O_2 is removed from the hemoglobin and taken up by the cells through diffusion in the capillaries. CO_2 leaves the cells and enters the bloodstream also through diffusion. Approximately 20% of the CO_2 will be dissolved in the blood plasma (Collins et al., 2015). In the presence of carbonic anhydrase, the remaining CO_2 combines with H_2O to briefly form carbonic acid (H_2CO_3), which quickly breaks into an H^+ and HCO_3^-. The H^+ binds with the hemoglobin and is transported to the lungs. There, the H^+ is removed from the hemoglobin, and the chemical process is reversed; the resulting CO_2 is excreted by the lungs, and the H_2O is excreted by the kidneys. The process is described by this chemical equation (Kamel & Halperin, 2017):

$$CO_2 + H_2O \leftrightarrow H_2CO_3 \leftrightarrow H^+ + HCO_3^{-\omega}$$

Hemoglobin's ability to carry O_2, its *affinity*, depends primarily on three factors (Collins et al., 2015):

- Acidity (blood pH)
- Temperature
- Presence of CO_2 (PCO_2)

Affinity changes are illustrated by the oxygen dissociation curve (Figure 1.1). As any or all of these three factors increase, the curve shifts to right indicating that hemoglobin loses its affinity for O_2. Conversely, as the factors decrease, the curve

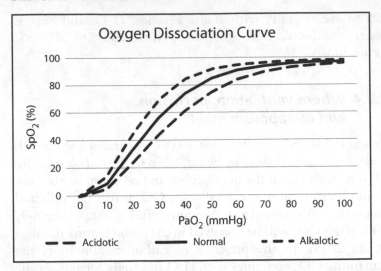

Figure 1.1 Oxygen dissociation curve.

shifts to the left, indicating that hemoglobin increases its affinity for O_2. When the body is in homeostasis, hemoglobin releases its O_2 in the (relatively) acidic, warm, high-CO_2 environment of the cellular capillaries, and takes on O_2 in the (relatively) basic, cool, low-CO_2 environment of the alveolar capillaries (Collins et al., 2015).

If any or all of the factors are deranged, it affects the ability of hemoglobin to properly perfuse the cells. If the body becomes acidotic, hyperthermic, or hypercarbic, hemoglobin cannot bind with O_2, which causes the cells to become hypoxic and switch to anaerobic metabolism. This further increases the acidosis and decreases the amount of CO_2 being generated. Since O_2 cannot replace the H^+ being held by the hemoglobin, less CO_2 can be exhaled from the lungs even though excess CO_2 is being generated. HCO_3^- is used to buffer (i.e., neutralize) the excess acids (Schlichtig & Bowles, 1994; Ward, 2011). This reduces the amount of HCO_3^- available at the lungs, further reducing the body's ability to remove the bound

H^+ and circulating CO_2, thus further aggravating the acidosis (Kartal et al., 2011).

Similarly, if the body becomes basic, hypothermic, or hypo-carbic, hemoglobin cannot release O_2. This results in hypoxia. The resulting acids are buffered by the excess circulating HCO_3^-. Less CO_2 is produced due to the cellular hypoxia, and the H^+ that is produced from CO_2 cannot be carried away as the hemoglobin has no available "slots" due to its "hoard-ing" O_2. This reduces the amount of CO_2 exhaled from the lungs (Collins et al., 2015).

1.4 HOW CAPNOGRAPHY WORKS

CO_2 is measured by shining an infrared beam through a sample of exhaled gases onto a sensor (Figure 1.2). CO_2 will absorb a particular frequency of light. By comparing the amount of light received versus transmitted, the amount of CO_2 in the sample can be determined.

The measurement can be performed in the display unit or at the airway. Side-stream capnography, where exhaled gas is pulled into the sensor in the display unit via a vacuum pump, is the most common. This allows measurements from patients with an intact gag reflex, using a modified nasal cannula, as well as from patients with advanced airways (i.e., endotracheal

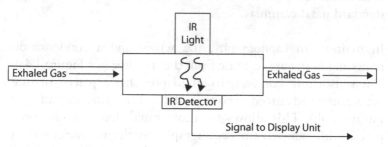

Figure 1.2 Measuring CO_2.

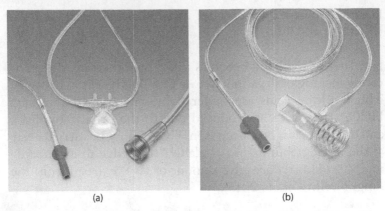

(a)   (b)

Figure 1.3 (a) Side-stream capnography nasal cannula and (b) in-line
adapter.

tubes or supraglottic airways) using an in-line adapter (see
Figure 1.3). This system has the advantage of simplicity but at
the cost of some reliability due to its narrow lumen, which may
become obstructed by condensation or secretions. There is also
a slight time lag between the exhalation and the measurement
due to the gas having to travel from the sampling site to the
display unit. On nasal sensors with O_2 delivery capability
(Figure 1.3a), note that O_2 is delivered through holes at the
base of the sensor; the prongs are part of the sampling system.
This limits the O_2 flow rate to 5 l/min versus 6 l/min through
standard nasal cannulas.

In mainstream capnography, the sensor and a condensation
removing heater are separate from the monitor (see Figure 1.4a).
The sensor unit connects to an adapter that is placed in-line
between an advanced airway and the breathing circuit (see
Figure 1.4b). This allows for more rapid detection as com-
pared with side-stream capnography as the measurement is
not delayed by having to draw a sample through a tube, but

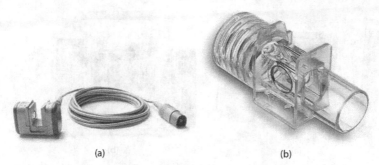

(a)   (b)

Figure 1.4 (a) Mainstream capnography sensor and (b) airway adapter.

Source: Both pictures ©2023 Koninklijke Philips N. V.

this method cannot be used for patients without advanced airways such as endotracheal tubes or supraglottic airways (e.g., patients with an intact gag reflex).

The results of the calculations (i.e., capnography) are displayed to the provider in two components:

- *Capnometry*: The most recently calculated $ETCO_2$ value and the number of ventilations (i.e., breaths) per minute.
- *Capnogram*: A continuous waveform that shows the amount of CO_2 present in real time.

Capnography devices combine both capnometry and a capnogram on a single display (Figure 1.5a). Many monitors combine several functions into a single screen, thus allowing the provider to monitor cardiac function, pulse oximetry, and capnography via a single device and screen (Figure 1.5b).

1.5 INTERPRETING CAPNOMETRY

The capnometry section of the display shows the breaths per minute and the most recent $ETCO_2$ value (see the bottom-left corner of Figure 1.5a). The normal $ETCO_2$ range is 35–45 mmHg or 4.6–6.0 kPa (Akca, 2011).

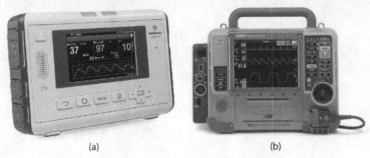

(a) (b)

Figure 1.5 (a) Capnography device and (b) multiparameter device.

Abnormal low $ETCO_2$ measurements indicate that less CO_2 is being exhaled than expected. This can be the result of

- Hypoxia reducing the amount of CO_2 being created.
- Hypometabolic states reducing the amount of CO_2 being created.
- Hyperventilation depleting the body of H^+.
- Metabolic acidosis, which reduces the amount of HCO_3^- available to extract H^+ from the bloodstream.
- A combination of all of these.

Abnormal high $ETCO_2$ measurements indicate that more CO_2 is being exhaled than expected. This can be the result of

- Hypermetabolic states increasing the amount of CO_2 being generated.
- Respiratory abnormalities causing CO_2 retention.
- Both

The following chapters describe specific conditions and how they are reflected in capnometry. Chapter 10 provides a table of differential diagnosis for different capnometry combinations.

1.6 INTERPRETING CAPNOGRAMS

The remainder of the capnography display is the capnogram (see the bottom of Figure 1.5b). This waveform shows the amount of CO_2 in the gas sample (expressed as a partial pressure) over time. The respiratory baseline (see Figure 1.6), from points A to B, represents exhalation from the anatomic dead space, i.e., parts of the respiratory system that do not take part in gas exchange such as the trachea and mainstem bronchi; this should be zero. The expiratory upstroke, from points B to C, represents a mix of dead space and alveolar exhalation. The alveolar plateau, from points C to D, represents alveolar exhalation, with the end point D representing the $ETCO_2$ value. The inhalation downstroke, from points D to E, represents inhalation of gas that is nearly free of CO_2 (Ward & Yealy, 1998).

The waveform changes based on the changes in the patient's ventilations. Changes in the patient's inspiratory-expiratory (I:E) ratio (i.e., the ratio of inhalation time versus expiration time) or CO_2 retention may change the respiratory baseline. Obstructions in the lower airways will change the morphology of the expiratory upstroke. An inability to ventilate the lower alveoli will change the alveolar plateau.

Cardiac rhythm and capnogram timescales are different on devices that display both. Cardiac rhythms are displayed at

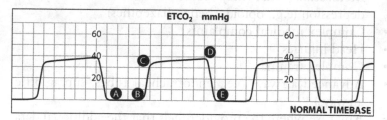

Figure 1.6 Normal capnogram with key points.

Source: From Ward & Yealy (1998).

25 mm/s, whereas the capnogram waveforms are displayed at 6.25–12.5 mm/s (depending on the screen size and manufacturer). This allows multiple breaths to be displayed on a screen at the same time. When printing the cardiac rhythm and the corresponding capnogram on the same "strip", devices will use the cardiogram's time scale, which will "stretch" the capnogram, but allow a detailed analysis of what the cardiac and respiratory functions were doing at any given point in time.

The following chapters describe specific conditions and how they are reflected in capnogram. Chapter 9 provides an algorithmic approach to evaluating and interpreting capnograms.

1.7 WHEN TO USE CAPNOGRAPHY

Primarily due to the expense of the sensors (US$10 each), capnography is not recommended to be used as a "fifth vital sign" (after pulse rate, ventilatory rate, blood pressure, and pulse oximetry). Capnography is strongly recommended for patients who need more in-depth evaluation and management, including but not limited to patients with

- Respiratory complaints
- Cardiac complaints
- Altered mental status
- Medication/drug overdoses
- Medications that may cause central nervous system depression (e.g., opioids, benzodiazepines)
- Complex medical complaints
- Head injuries
- Complex trauma
- Advanced airways (i.e., endotracheal tubes, supraglottic airways)
- Any case where the provider feels that the additional data will be of benefit

Specific indications are discussed in the following chapters.

1.8 DIAGNOSING EQUIPMENT PROBLEMS

The DOPE mnemonic used for diagnosing airway adjunct errors can also be used, with minor modifications, for diagnosing problems with capnography equipment.

- *Dislodgement*: Check that the nasal sensor is not moved out of position. Ensure that an airway attached to an in-line or mainstream sensor has not been dislodged. Ensure that the sensor tube or cable is correctly and securely attached to the capnography monitor.

- *Occlusion*: Check that the tubing from a side-stream sensor to the device is uncoiled and not pinched or otherwise mechanically compromised. The narrow lumen of side stream sensors is prone to clogging with condensation or secretions; it may be necessary to replace the sensor. Similarly, ensure that the window on a mainstream sensor has not been occluded by condensation, medications, or secretions.

- *Placement*: Ensure that the nasal sensor is properly placed. It may be difficult or impossible to get reliable measurements on patients with inadequate upper dentation. Ensure that an in-line or mainstream sensor is properly attached and that the attached airway is properly placed.

- *Equipment*: Verify that the selected sensor is correctly sized. For in-line sensors, it may be necessary to use a pediatric, infant, neonatal sensor to reduce the amount of dead space in the circuit. Ensure that the capnography monitor is functioning correctly. First, try power cycling the device. If that does not work, it may be necessary to completely discontinue use of the capnography device until it can be inspected, calibrated, and/or repaired.

Consult the device's user manual for diagnostic information of the specific device.

1.9 STUDY QUESTIONS

1 What is ventilation? What is respiration? How are these represented on a capnography display?

2 How does CO_2 output relate to ventilation, perfusion, and metabolism?

3 What is the relationship between HCO_3^- and CO_2 output?

4 Name the segments of the capnogram. What does each represent? What does an abnormal presentation of each mean?

REFERENCES

Akca, O. (2011). Tissue- and organ-specific effects of carbon dioxide. In J. S. Gravenstein, M. B. Jaffe, N. Gravenstein, & D. A. Paulus (Eds.), *Capnography* (2nd ed., pp. 250–260). Cambridge University Press.

Choi, S. J., Ahn, H. J., Yang, M. K., Kim, C. S., Sim, W. S., Kim, J. A., Kang, J. G., Kim, J. K., & Kang, J. Y. (2010). Comparison of desaturation and resaturation response times between transmission and reflectance pulse oximeters. *Acta Anaesthesiologica Scandinavica*, 54(2). https://doi.org/10.1111/j.1399-6576.2009.02101.x

Collins, J. A., Rudenski, A., Gibson, J., Howard, L., & O'Driscoll, R. (2015). Relating oxygen partial pressure, saturation and content: The haemoglobin–oxygen dissociation curve. *Breathe*, 11(3), 194–201. https://doi.org/10.1183/20734735.001415

Kamel, K. S., & Halperin, M. L. (2017). *Fluid, Electrolyte, and Acid-Base Physiology* (5th ed.). Elsevier.

Kartal, M., Eray, O., Rinnert, S., Goksu, E., Bektas, F., & Eken, C. (2011). $ETCO_2$: A predictive tool for excluding metabolic disturbances in nonintubated patients. *American Journal of Emergency Medicine*, 29(1), 65–69. https://doi.org/10.1016/j.ajem.2009.08.001

NAEMT & ACS. (2019). *PHTLS: Prehospital Trauma Life Support* (9th ed.). Jones Bartlett.

Schlichtig, R., & Bowles, S. A. (1994). Distinguishing between aerobic and anaerobic appearance of dissolved CO_2 in intestine during low flow. *Journal of Applied Physiology*, 76(6). https://doi.org/10.1152/jappl.1994.76.6.2443

Ward, K. R. (2011). The physiological basis for capnometric monitoring in shock. In J. S. Gravenstein, M. B. Jaffe, N. Gravenstein, & D. A. Paulus (Eds.), *Capnography* (2nd ed., pp. 231–238). Cambridge University Press.

Ward, K. R., & Yealy, D. M. (1998). End-tidal carbon dioxide monitoring in emergency medicine, Part 1: Basic principles. *Academic Emergency Medicine, 5*(6), 628–636. https://doi.org/10.1111/j.1553-2712.1998.tb02473.x

NOTES

AIRWAY MANAGEMENT

This chapter examines how capnography can help with managing patients with advanced airways.

2.1 AIRWAY VERIFICATION

A constant worry when using an advanced airway is ensuring that the airway is correctly placed. An incorrectly placed airway, especially an endotracheal tube, can result in a patient not receiving oxygen for an extended period, with potentially lethal results. This worry is closely followed by the concern that the airway remains in place. Capnography is superior to (but does not completely replace) other airway placement verification methods as it provides objective proof of airway placement.

After placing the airway, place an in-line sensor on the airway (see Figure 1.3b) and then connect the bag-valve-mask or ventilator to the sensor. Ventilate the patient, while auscultating as usual, and observe the capnography display. If square waveforms with non-zero $ETCO_2$ measurements are observed consistently over several breaths, the airway is in the trachea (Donald & Paterson, 2006; Silvestri et al., 2017). One or two waveforms may be observed in esophageal intubations due to the presence of small amounts of CO_2. Note that auscultation is still required to ensure that an endotracheal tube is not

DOI: 10.1201/9781003491576-2

placed into the right mainstem bronchus. Consider attaching a print-out of the capnogram to the patient care report as proof that the airway was correctly placed.

If an endotracheal tube is placed into the esophagus, or if a supraglottic airway is not correctly sealed around the tracheal opening, the waveform will be flat and the $ETCO_2$ measurements will be zero or close to it. Presentations of various endotracheal tube failures are described in the next section.

After each patient movement (e.g., on to the stretcher and from the stretcher to the hospital bed), a non-zero $ETCO_2$ reading combined with a square waveform with each ventilation verifies that the airway is not dislodged or otherwise compromised. Consider attaching a print-out of the capnogram for each time the patient is moved to the patient care report to prove that the airway remained patent at each checkpoint.

2.2 ENDOTRACHEAL TUBE MANAGEMENT

A capnogram with an inverted V appearance may indicate a kinked tube (Figure 2.1) (Ward & Yealy, 1998).

A capnogram with a rounded appearance and a normopneic rate may indicate a tube with a deflated cuff (Figure 2.2) (Ward & Yealy, 1998).

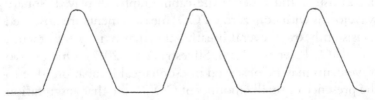

Figure 2.1 Capnogram indicating a kinked endotracheal tube.

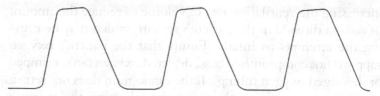

Figure 2.2 Capnogram indicating a leaking endotracheal tube cuff.

A capnogram that suddenly goes to zero may indicate that the tube has become dislodged or clogged. It may also indicate ventilator failure or that the patient has become apneic.

2.3 SEDATED/PARALYZED OR ANESTHETIZED PATIENTS

Patients that have been sedated and paralyzed to support rapid sequence intubation (RSI), or have been anesthetized, may attempt to inhale during exhalation, which is observable in the capnogram, as shown in Figure 2.3. This waveform, sometimes referred to as a "curare cleft", indicates that the patient may be

- Gasping due to hypercarbia (i.e., $ETCO_2$ greater than 45 mmHg) or hypoxia
- Gasping in pain
- Suffering thoracic compression (e.g., provider leaning on the patient while reaching for equipment) (Gravenstein, 2011)

Before administering additional medication, check the $ETCO_2$ measurement; if it is on the high end of normal, consider

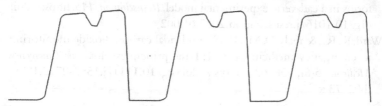

Figure 2.3 Patient fighting mechanical ventilation.

increasing the ventilation rate or volume to reduce the amount of carbon dioxide in the patient's system, which may be causing the attempts to inhale. Ensure that the patient's oxygen supply is not compromised (e.g., depleted oxygen tank, crimped or dislodged oxygen tubing). If the capnogram does not return to a square waveform, then consider adjusting the patient's medication (Gravenstein, 2011; Ward & Yealy, 1998).

2.4 STUDY QUESTIONS

1 How does a non-zero $ETCO_2$ measurement assure the provider that an advanced airway is correctly placed?

2 Why is the inspiratory downstroke sharply sloped with a leaky endotracheal tube balloon?

3 What vital sign may help in diagnosing a notched alveolar plateau? Why?

REFERENCES

Donald, M. J., & Paterson, B. (2006). End tidal carbon dioxide monitoring in prehospital and retrieval medicine: A review. *Emergency Medicine Journal, 23*(9). https://doi.org/10.1136/emj.2006.037184

Gravenstein, J. S. (2011). Clinical perspectives. In D. A. Gravenstien, J.S. Jaffe, M. B. Gravenstien, N. Paulus (Eds.), *Capnography* (2nd ed.). Cambridge University Press.

Silvestri, S., Ladde, J. G., Brown, J. F., Roa, J.V., Hunter, C., Ralls, G. A., & Papa, L. (2017). Endotracheal tube placement confirmation: 100% sensitivity and specificity with sustained four-phase capnographic waveforms in a cadaveric experimental model. *Resuscitation, 115*. https://doi.org/10.1016/j.resuscitation.2017.01.002

Ward, K. R., & Yealy, D. M. (1998). End-tidal carbon dioxide monitoring in emergency medicine, Part 1: Basic principles. *Academic Emergency Medicine, 5*(6), 628–636. https://doi.org/10.1111/j.1553-2712.1998.tb02473.x

NOTES

NOTES

RESPIRATORY EMERGENCIES

This chapter describes how capnography can be used to diagnose and manage patients with respiratory emergencies.

3.1 ARTIFICIAL VENTILATION MANAGEMENT

It is important to remember that oxygen is a medication. It must be administered in amounts and with timing that is titrated to the desired effect. Different patients with different conditions need different rates and volumes. A capnography-based management approach adjusts the rate and/or volume to keep the patient's $ETCO_2$ within a range that is appropriate for the patient's condition, while maintaining oxygenation (Cooper et al., 2013). Chapters 7 and 8 prevent hyper- or hypoventilation in the patient (Davis, 2011; Rozycki et al., 1998).

Patients with respiratory distress ($ETCO_2$ greater than 50 mmHg) (Krauss & Hess, 2007) or respiratory arrest, including those undergoing rapid sequence intubation, who do not fit under any of the management categories covered in this or other chapters, should be ventilated as follows:

- *$ETCO_2$ between 30 and 45 mmHg*: Ventilate at 10 to 12 breaths per minute to maintain $ETCO_2$ between 30 and 45 mmHg with $SpO_2 \geq 94\%$ (AHA, 2020).

DOI: 10.1201/9781003491576-3

- *ETCO$_2$ less than 30 mmHg*: Ventilate to maintain SpO$_2$ ≥ 94%. Never withhold ventilations. If this is insufficient to restore normocarbia (i.e., ETCO$_2$ between 35 and 45 mmHg), reduce the ventilatory volume while ensuring that the patient is being properly oxygenated (Davis, 2011). These ETCO$_2$ measurements may indicate perfusion or metabolic issues that may not be correctable through ventilation (Cooper et al., 2013; Doppmann et al., 2021). "The maintenance of pH balance requires a finely coordinated effort by the brain, renal, respiratory, and cardiovascular systems. These systems are very efficient at managing metabolic derangements and overriding the respiratory system to correct a metabolic abnormality should be done with extreme caution" (Diskin, 2022). See Chapters 6 and 7.

- *ETCO$_2$ greater than 45 mmHg*: Ventilate the patient at 12 to 20 breaths per minute until eucapnia (i.e., ETCO$_2$ between 35 and 45 mmHg) is reached. Avoid SpO$_2$ values greater than 99%.

3.2 RESPIRATORY ACIDOSIS

Respiratory acidosis occurs when the patient is not ventilating sufficiently to exhale enough CO$_2$ from the lungs to maintain the body's acid/base balance. Respiratory acidosis is a diagnostic sign, not a diagnosis, which results from a variety of conditions that reduce the minute volume of ventilations (i.e., the volume of air inhaled/exhaled per minute). This can result from pain (e.g., broken ribs, burns), airway obstruction (e.g., bronchospasm, foreign-body obstruction, pneumonia), or central nervous system (CNS) disturbance (e.g., drug/medication overdose, cerebral vascular accident, traumatic brain injury).

Respiratory acidosis can further be divided into acute and chronic, with chronic defined as acidosis lasting long enough for the kidneys to produce extra bicarbonate (greater than 24 hours) (Boysen & Isenberg, 2011; Kamel & Halperin, 2017).

Respiratory acidosis manifests as $ETCO_2$ measurements greater than 45 mmHg, with ventilatory rates dependent upon the mechanism of the respiratory disruption. Central nervous system disturbances from opiate overdoses or traumatic brain injury may present with bradypnea (i.e., ventilatory rate less than 10 breaths per minute), with normal tidal volumes. Obstructive disruptions may present with normopnea or mild tachypnea (i.e., a ventilatory rate greater than 20 breaths per minute), with accessory muscle use and reduced tidal volumes. Pain and thoracic trauma may present with severe tachypnea with low tidal volumes. Treatment is centered on either correcting the cause (e.g., medication for bronchospasm or opiate overdose), mitigating the cause (e.g., pain reduction measures), or providing artificial ventilation (e.g., bag-valve-mask or mechanical ventilation) to provide normal tidal volumes (Boysen & Isenberg, 2011; Kamel & Halperin, 2017).

Acute respiratory acidosis can result in anxiety, dyspnea, confusion, and/or psychosis. Chronic respiratory acidosis can cause sleep disturbances, memory loss, daytime somnolence, altered mental status, coordination impairment, and/or motor dysfunctions. Hypercarbia causes dilation of cerebral arterioles, which is potentially dangerous in traumatic brain injury and stroke patients (see Chapter 6). Hypercarbia can increase catecholamines, which can be harmful to patients with cardiac dysfunctions (see Section 4.3). Hypercarbia leads to a build-up of unbuffered H^+ ions, leading to these ions binding to various intracellular proteins resulting in changes in their charge, shape, and/or function (Boysen & Isenberg, 2011; Kamel & Halperin, 2017). This can lead to effects such as decreased cardiac contractility, central nervous system depression, and glucose intolerance (Boysen & Isenberg, 2011).

In bradypnea, the patient does not breathe fast enough to remove CO_2. The patient has a ventilatory rate of less than

10 breaths per minute, with gradually increasing $ETCO_2$ measurements. The patient should be artificially ventilated as described in Section 3.1.

Respiratory acidosis can occur in patients who are normopneic or mildly tachypneic (10 to 30 breaths per minute) when they have insufficient tidal volume to excrete sufficient CO_2. This may be the result of a thoracic trauma (e.g., fractured rib) or abdominal pain that restricts the patient's ability to ventilate. Treatment is focused on correcting or mitigating the patient's condition and monitoring for respiratory failure (Section 3.12) or arrest (Section 3.13).

In severe tachypnea, the patient breathes very fast, more than 30 breaths per minute, which results in incomplete exhalation, leaving most (if not all) of the alveoli filled with CO_2 (Figure 3.1). Note the capnogram's almost sinusoidal (i.e., rounded) appearance. The patient's $PaCO_2$ will be much greater than the displayed $ETCO_2$ since the patient never completely empties the alveoli, thus the peak CO_2 value is never reached (Gravenstein, 2011). Treatment is focused on mitigating the patient's condition while monitoring for impending respiratory failure (Section 3.12) or arrest (Section 3.13).

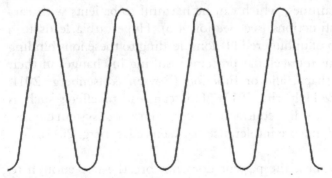

Figure 3.1 Severe tachypnea capnogram.

3.3 RESPIRATORY ALKALOSIS

Respiratory alkalosis occurs when the patient, through hyperventilation, exhales too much CO_2. Hyperventilation can result from numerous causes, including hypoxia (e.g., high altitude, shock), chest receptor stimulation (e.g., thoracic trauma), central nervous system stimulation (e.g., fever, intracranial bleed, pain, anxiety), medications/drugs/hormones (e.g., xanthines, salicylates, catecholamines), sepsis, liver failure, and pregnancy. Artificial ventilation at a too high rate may result in respiratory alkalosis. It is a frequent finding in heart failure and early respiratory failure (Boysen & Isenberg, 2011; Kamel & Halperin, 2017).

Signs and symptoms, in addition to those of the underlying illness, may include dizziness, confusion, and seizures resulting from decreased cerebral blood flow. Patients with heart disease may experience dysrhythmias as hemoglobin is unable to unload oxygen due to alkalosis. Capnography will indicate tachypnea with $ETCO_2$ measurements less than 30 mmHg (Boysen & Isenberg, 2011).

The treatment is to improve or maintain oxygenation between 94% and 99%, and resolve or mitigate the underlying disease process. The minute ventilations of artificially ventilated patients should be adjusted with the goal being to bring the $ETCO_2$ into the 30–35 mmHg range while maintaining oxygenation; see Section 3.1.

3.4 HYPERVENTILATION SYNDROME

Hyperventilation syndrome is a condition where the patient ventilates faster than the body needs to meet metabolic or respiratory demands. It typically manifests as a combination of tachypnea with numbness, tingling, and/or carpopedal spasms, along with a history of an anxiety- or stress-inducing event. These symptoms may be anxiety-inducing themselves, thus perpetuating the syndrome. These patients will present with $SpO_2 \geq 94\%$ (i.e., adequate oxygenation), tachycardia, tachypnea with full deep breaths having square waveforms, and $ETCO_2$ measurements less than 30 mmHg that can be as low as 15 mmHg (Boysen & Isenberg, 2011).

When left unchecked, the patient may become unconscious or suffer dysrhythmias. It is important to get a thorough medical history to exclude more serious causes for the patient's hyperventilation (e.g., traumatic brain injury, drug/medication overdose). An electrocardiogram should be obtained to rule out cardiovascular etiologies. Hyperventilation syndrome should be a diagnosis of exclusion (i.e., all other diagnoses have been ruled out before settling on this diagnosis).

The treatment, and challenge, is to help the patient get their ventilatory rate back into a healthy range. The capnography monitor can help by using it for biofeedback. Tell the patient that they need to either reduce their ventilatory rate or increase their $ETCO_2$ measurement. In many cases, the patient will be able to "adjust" their ventilations to improve their status. If nothing else, the exercise may distract the patient from both the anxiety trigger and their discomfort, which may improve their ventilatory status (Meckley, 2009; Meuret, 2011).

3.5 VENTILATION/PERFUSION (V/Q) MISMATCH

Ventilation/Perfusion (V/Q) mismatch occurs when the lungs can inhale a normal tidal volume, but gas exchange is compromised. This can be the result of compromised pulmonary circulation (e.g., pulmonary embolism), alveolar damage or dysfunction, or toxic exposure (e.g., carbon monoxide). The patient's lungs may be clear and equal to auscultation, and the patient's signs and symptoms (low O_2 saturation and dyspnea) are not specific. The patient may not complain of chest pain. Electrocardiography may indicate strain or ischemia but will not be diagnostic.

Capnography will not generally aid in diagnosing the cause of the mismatch, but it may aid in its detection. A patient with a V/Q mismatch will present with tachypnea and normal to low $ETCO_2$ on capnometry, reminiscent of hyperventilation syndrome. The patient will breathe faster to make up for the decreased exchange by increasing the amount of air available for exchange.

None of the tools available to field providers (capnography, electrocardiography, pulse oximetry), alone or in combination, can definitively diagnose either the presence or cause of a V/Q mismatch. The patient's history in combination with the signs of impaired perfusion should lead the provider to include this in their differential diagnosis.

3.6 BRONCHOSPASM

It is important to differentiate bronchospasm from other causes of respiratory difficulty to ensure that treatments are used appropriately for both the problem and the patient. While patient's history may provide clues (e.g., asthma, emphysema), diagnosis, especially in the field, tends to rely on auscultation. This presents problems for the provider as it may be difficult to hear or interpret lung sounds due to (among other complications) patient habitus, ambient noise, or patient ventilations that are too shallow to create the necessary turbulence.

Bronchospasm can be rapidly identified via capnography. A patient with active bronchospasm will have a waveform with a sloping expiratory upstroke, as opposed to a normal nearly vertical expiratory upstroke, often referred to as a "shark fin";

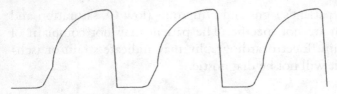

Figure 3.2 Bronchospasm capnogram.

see Figure 3.2. This is caused by prolonged exhalation due to constriction. The inspiratory downstroke may also be sloped, rather than nearly vertical, due to difficulty in exhaling from the bottom of the alveolar tree. These patients will typically be tachypneic and hypercarbic (Yaron et al., 1996; You et al., 1994).

If the patient responds well to treatment, their capnogram will gradually return to a more normal appearance. When combined with the patient expressing symptom relief, this gives the provider reassurance that the treatment is effective, and the patient's emergency is (for the moment) under control.

Conversely, increasing $ETCO_2$ measurements and a decreasing I:E ratio indicate that the patient is progressing (or has progressed) into respiratory failure (see Section 3.12). This is the result of fatigue from having to use accessory muscles to force gas from the lungs, which is normally a passive process. The I:E ratio decreases as the passive expiratory process can no longer provide sufficient pressure to empty the lungs, thus prematurely ending the expiratory phase. This may also lead to breath stacking (see Section 3.10).

3.7 CONGESTIVE HEART FAILURE

In congestive heart failure, the heart does not pump effectively, causing blood to back up into the lungs. When the pressure reaches a threshold, plasma and other fluids in the bloodstream are forced into the alveoli, leading to a decrease in gas exchange, along with the patient experiencing dyspnea.

The challenge for providers is differentiating between congestive heart failure and restrictive etiologies. The patient's history will provide some clues. It is common to use auscultation, but as already noted, it can be difficult to hear and interpret lung sounds.

In congestive heart failure, the capnogram will have a near-normal appearance, with nearly square waveforms. This is because there is no obstruction in the gas flow into and out of the lungs, in contrast with asthma and chronic obstructive pulmonary diseases (see Section 3.6). Congestive heart failure patients will be tachypneic and hypocarbic, resulting in respiratory alkalosis (see Section 3.3) (Boysen & Isenberg, 2011), proportionately to the number of alveoli that cannot be ventilated. These signs, along with the patient's history, cardiography, and low SpO_2, increase the provider's confidence in a working diagnosis of congestive heart failure.

3.8 MUCUS PLUGGING

Various disease processes can result in mucus build-up in the lungs. This may cause bronchioles to become transiently plugged. A patient with mucus plugging may present with a caponogram, as shown in Figure 3.3. The plateau in the inspiratory downstroke is caused by mucus plugs that are dislodged by pressure behind the plug or a cough-like spasm, which dislodges blockages, leading to a brief mini-exhalation. Depending on the degree of mucus build-up, the patient may show a decrease in $ETCO_2$ (less than 35 mmHg), low O_2 saturation, and dyspnea.

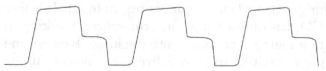

Figure 3.3 Mucus plugging capnogram.

3.9 COLLAPSED LUNG

A collapsed lung may result from air leaking into the pleural space (pneumothorax), blood leaking into the pleural space (hemothorax), or damage to the lung from a disease process (e.g., lung cancer). Auscultation will reveal severely diminished or absent lung sounds on the affected side, but ambient noise conditions may make auscultation difficult or unreliable. The patient's signs and symptoms (low O_2 saturation and dyspnea) by themselves are not diagnostic, lacking a convincing history (e.g., recent thoracic trauma).

The capnography of a patient with only one working lung, or a collapsing lung, will show tachypnea with low to normal $ETCO_2$ measurements (Lee et al., 2021). Again, this constellation of signs, without a history of thoracic trauma or a medical condition that predisposes the patient to lung collapse, is not specific, but should cause a collapsed lung to be added to the provider's differential diagnosis.

3.10 BREATH STACKING

Breath stacking typically occurs when exhalations are restricted, resulting in incomplete removal of CO_2 from the lungs, which leads to the next exhalation not starting from zero. This condition is apparent on the capnogram as a stair-step pattern (Thompson & Jaffe, 2005), as shown in Figure 3.4. The respiratory baseline does not return to zero, and each complex is more elevated than the previous. This can result from rebreathing or auto-PEEP (positive end-expiratory pressure).

Rebreathing occurs when the patient begins to inhale before exhaled CO_2 has diffused into the atmosphere, resulting in the patient bringing excess CO_2 into the lungs. Rebreathing is usually the result of oxygen delivery equipment failure, such as oxygen supply interruptions to a continuous positive

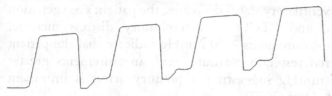

Figure 3.4 Breath stacking capnogram.

airway pressure (CPAP) or non-rebreather mask (Thompson & Jaffe, 2005). This decreases the amount of O_2 available for exchange and increases the amount of CO_2 that the body needs to excrete. When left unchecked, the patient will eventually suffer the effects of both hypoxia and hypercarbia.

Auto-PEEP occurs when the lungs do not have sufficient time to completely exhale before the next inhalation occurs. This is most often the result of ventilator settings (Laghi & Goyal, 2012), but can also occur with bronchospasm patients in (or near) respiratory failure.

3.11 PREMATURE INHALATION (GASPING)

Spontaneously breathing patients may take a shallow breath (or gasp) in the middle of exhalation. This manifests as a notched capnogram, similar to those seen in intubated patients (see Figure 2.3). This occurs for similar reasons, specifically due to hypoxia or pain. Consider adjusting the patient's oxygen flow or pain medications.

3.12 RESPIRATORY FAILURE

It is important to recognize a patient that is nearing or (worse) in respiratory failure. Respiratory failure indicates that the patient is tiring and cannot ventilate adequately to support respiration. In the early stages, the patient may hyperventilate, with $ETCO_2$ measurements less than 30 mmHg, to maintain oxygenation (Boysen & Isenberg, 2011). As the patient's ventilatory status decreases, the patient's oxygenation decreases, and $ETCO_2$ and respiratory distress increase. $ETCO_2$ measurements ≥ 70 mmHg indicate that the patient has entered respiratory failure, with measurements greater than 80 mmHg suggesting respiratory arrest is imminent (Krauss & Hess, 2007).

Having said this, it is important to note that chronic obstructive pulmonary disease (COPD) patients may have baseline (i.e., normal for the patient) $ETCO_2$ measurements greater than 45 mmHg. In this patient population, an $ETCO_2$ measurement greater than 60 mmHg alone, without respiratory distress, may not necessarily indicate impending respiratory failure (Diskin, 2022). Treat the patient, not the numbers.

3.13 RESPIRATORY ARREST

Ideally, impending respiratory arrest is recognized visually and early; the providers actively watch the patient and are able to react instantly if the patient stops breathing. Unfortunately, providers are often distracted with other patient care necessities, and patient ventilation may be hard to visualize due to shallow depth, slow rate, body habitus, or clothing. Capnography continuously monitors the patient's ventilations, so apnea can be detected (and an alarm generated) within a few seconds, whereas it can take pulse oximetry more than 60 seconds to react to apnea (Cacho et al., 2010). Immediate action, including capnography-guided artificial ventilations (see Section 3.1), is required to save the patient's life.

3.14 AIRWAY OBSTRUCTION

Full airway obstruction does not require capnography to diagnose; it will be apparent from the patient exhibiting the "Universal" Choking Sign or the inability to mechanically ventilate the patient. Partial upper airway obstructions usually result in inspiratory stridor; again, capnography is not needed to diagnose these.

Partial lower airway obstructions between the vocal cords and the carina may not present with an audible stridor. A significant obstruction may present in the capnogram, as shown in Figure 2.1. The prolonged expiratory upstroke and inspiratory downstroke result from the increased effort necessary for the patient to ventilate around the obstruction.

Obstructions below the carina may result in dyspnea and decreased $ETCO_2$ measurements, in proportion to the airway volume obstructed, resulting from decreased ventilation of the affected lung. The waveform will be essentially normal.

3.15 STUDY QUESTIONS

1 Why is it desirable to maintain $ETCO_2$ between 30 and 35 mmHg versus the normal range of 35–45 mmHg during artificial ventilations?

2 What are the signs and symptoms of respiratory acidosis and respiratory alkalosis?

3 What does a "shark fin" waveform indicate? Why? How can the waveform tell us if our treatment is effective?

4 How can capnography help differentiate between congestive and obstructive etiologies of dyspnea?

REFERENCES

AHA. (2020). *Advanced Cardiovascular Life Support*. American Heart Association.

Boysen, P. G., & Isenberg, A. V. (2011). Acid-base balance and diagnosis of disorders. In J. S. Gravenstein, M. B. Jaffe, N. Gravenstein, & D. A. Paulus (Eds.), *Capnography* (2nd ed.). Cambridge University Press.

Cacho, G., Pérez-Calle, J. L., Barbado, A., Lledó, J. L., Ojea, R., & Fernández-Rodríguez, C. M. (2010). Capnography is superior to pulse oximetry for the detection of respiratory depression during colonoscopy. *Revista Espanola de Enfermedades Digestivas*, *102*(2), 86–89. https://doi.org/10.4321/S1130-01082010000200003

Cooper, C. J., Kraatz, J. J., Kubiak, D. S., Kessel, J. W., & Barnes, S. L. (2013). Utility of prehospital quantitative end tidal CO_2? *Prehospital and Disaster Medicine*, *28*(2), 87–93. https://doi.org/10.1017/S1049023X12001768

Davis, D. P. (2011). Capnography as a guide to ventilation in the field. In D. A. Gravenstein, J. S. Jaffe, M. B. Gravenstein, N. Paulus (Eds.), *Capnography* (2nd ed.). Cambridge University Press.

Diskin, F. J. (2022). *Personal Correspondence*.

Doppmann, P., Meuli, L., Sollid, S. J. M., Filipovic, M., Knapp, J., Exadaktylos, A., Albrecht, R., & Pietsch, U. (2021). End-tidal to arterial carbon dioxide gradient is associated with increased mortality in patients with traumatic brain injury: A retrospective observational study. *Scientific Reports*, *11*(1), 1–9. https://doi.org/10.1038/s41598-021-89913-x

Gravenstein, J. S. (2011). Clinical Perspectives. In D. A. Gravenstien, J. S. Jaffe, M. B. Gravenstien, N. Paulus (Eds.), *Capnography* (2nd ed.). Cambridge University Press.

Kamel, K. S., & Halperin, M. L. (2017). *Fluid, Electrolyte, and Acid-Base Physiology* (5th ed.). Elsevier.

Krauss, B., & Hess, D. R. (2007). Capnography for procedural sedation and analgesia in the emergency department. *Annals of Emergency Medicine*, *50*(2), 172–181. https://doi.org/10.1016/j.annemergmed.2006.10.016

Laghi, F., & Goyal, A. (2012). Auto-PEEP in respiratory failure. *Minerva Anestesiologica*, *78*(2), 201–221.

Lee, G. M., Kim, Y. W., Lee, S., Do, H. H., Seo, J. S., & Lee, J. H. (2021). End-tidal carbon dioxide monitoring for spontaneous pneumothorax. *Emergency Medicine International*, *2021*, 1–6. https://doi.org/10.1155/2021/9976543

Meckley, A. (2009). Balancing unbalanced breathing: The clinical use of capnographic biofeedback. *Biofeedback*, *41*(4), 183–187. https://doi.org/10.5298/1081-5937-41.4.02

Meuret, A. E. (2011). Biofeedback. In J. S. Gravenstein, M. B. Jaffee, N. Gravenstein, & D. A. Paulus (Eds.), *Capnography* (2nd ed.). Cambridge University Press.

Rozycki, H. J., Sysyn, G. D., Marshall, M. K., Malloy, R., & Wiswell, T. J. (1998). Mainstream end-tidal carbon dioxide monitoring in the neonatal intensive care unit. *Pediatrics*, *101*(4.1) 648–653. https://doi.org/10.1542/peds.101.4.648

Thompson, J. E., & Jaffe, M. B. (2005). Capnographic waveforms in the mechanically ventilated patient. *Respiratory Care*, *50*(1), 100–109.

Yaron, M., Padyk, P., Hutsinpiller, M., & Cairns, C. B. (1996). Utility of the expiratory capnogram in the assessment of bronchospasm. *Annals of Emergency Medicine*, *28*(4), 403–407.

You, B., Peslin, R., Duvivier, C., Vu, V. D., & Grilliat, J. P. (1994). Expiratory capnography in asthma: Evaluation of various shape indices. *European Respiratory Journal*, *7*(2), 318–323. https://doi.org/10.1183/09031936.94.07020318

NOTES

4

CARDIAC EMERGENCIES

Electrocardiography is the primary diagnostic tool in cardiac emergencies. Capnography provides data that help clarify the meaning of the electrocardiographic data to improve patient outcomes.

4.1 CARDIAC ARREST

Adequate cardio-pulmonary resuscitation (CPR) is necessary to sustain a patient's life during cardiac arrest. CPR must be initiated quickly and efficiently to give the patient their best chance for survival. Key to this is ensuring that each member of the resuscitation team understands their specific role. To this end, the American Heart Association (AHA) has defined six roles and their specific responsibilities (AHA, 2020). The concept of high-performance resuscitation teams has been refined in the EMS milieu as pit crew CPR, where the role assignments are made at the beginning of each shift, thus each crew member can start their tasks once they "go over the wall" (i.e., arrive on scene).

The provider in the Airway role is responsible for ensuring that the capnography sensor is properly attached to the airway device in use. Capnography should be monitored during resuscitation regardless of the type of airway management devices being used (i.e., bag-valve-mask, supraglottic airway,

DOI: 10.1201/9781003491576-4

or endotracheal tube) (Carlson et al., 2021). Care needs to be taken when using a bag-valve-mask with an in-line sensor to ensure a good seal otherwise $ETCO_2$ measurements may not be reliable due to "contamination" with ambient air.

The provider in the Monitor/Defibrillator role must place the monitor in a position where it (ideally) can be viewed by the Airway, Compressor, and Team Leader providers. The Monitor/Defibrillator provider uses the $ETCO_2$ measurements to "coach" the Airway and Compressor providers. The Airway provider needs visibility into the $ETCO_2$ measurement to ensure that the device is properly placed (see Sections 2.1 and 2.2) and that ventilations are adequate. The Compressor provider needs visibility to ensure that compressions are being performed properly. The Team Leader needs the $ETCO_2$ measurements to provide a more detailed picture of the resuscitation efforts.

$ETCO_2$ measurements between 10 and 20 mmHg indicate that the body's processes are being supported at a level that will buy time for definitive treatments to be administered (AHA, 2020; Kodali & Urman, 2014; Meaney et al., 2013). Measurements less than 10 mmHg may indicate that ventilations are too frequent, or compressions are inadequate. Measurements greater than 20 mmHg may indicate ventilations are not frequent enough or compressions are inadequate.

There is evidence that the probability of a first shock successfully converting ventricular fibrillation (VFib) improves markedly if $ETCO_2$ measurements are above 11 mmHg (Chicote et al., 2019; Savastano et al., 2017). The theory is that a better perfused heart is more likely to respond to the shock than a poorly perfused (i.e., acidotic) heart. Providers may want to delay at least the first defibrillation attempt until $ETCO_2$ measurements exceed 11 mmHg.

Numerous studies have demonstrated that $ETCO_2$ measurements less than 10 mmHg despite adequate CPR and ventilations indicate that the patient has no chance of survival. This has not been incorporated into protocols because analyses have shown inconsistencies between the studies, which limit the ability to state with sufficient certainty that $ETCO_2$ less than 10 mmHg alone can be used to cease resuscitation efforts (Cone et al., 2011; Kodali & Urman, 2014; Touma & Davies, 2013). $ETCO_2$ measurements should be used in conjunction with other accepted indicators of futility after 20 minutes of Advanced Cardiovascular Life Support (e.g., no returns of spontaneous circulation at any time, no shockable rhythm at any time, pulseless electrical activity).

$ETCO_2$ measurements have been demonstrated to be lower than $PaCO_2$ in hypothermic arrest patients. The implication is that $ETCO_2$ measurements less than 10 mmHg must not be used as a criterion for terminating resuscitation efforts nor for excluding hypothermic patients from extracorporeal cardiopulmonary resuscitation (Darocha et al., 2022).

4.2 RETURN OF SPONTANEOUS CIRCULATION

The current AHA standards for CPR require that the provider check for return of spontaneous circulation (ROSC) only once every two minutes (AHA, 2020). This challenges the provider in determining if ROSC was achieved in-between checks, such as after defibrillation or administering a medication. A capnography monitor connected to an $ETCO_2$ sensor between an advanced airway and bag-valve-mask device can help us resolve this dilemma.

When a patient is in cardio–pulmonary arrest, perfusion is poor, even with excellent CPR (see Section 4.1). ROSC can be recognized by sudden and sustained measurements above 20 mmHg as perfusion dramatically improves, particularly in the heart and brain (AHA, 2020; Kodali & Urman, 2014). Readings above 50 mmHg are not uncommon. Ventilations should be adjusted to drive $ETCO_2$ measurements between 35 and 45 mmHg (see Section 3.1).

4.3 BRADYCARDIA

The AHA lists several possible causes of bradycardia, colloquially known as the "Hs and Ts" (AHA, 2020). One of the "Hs" is "Hydrogen Ions" or acidosis. Acidosis may result from either respiratory or metabolic causes. Correcting or mitigating the acidosis may mitigate or resolve the bradycardia (AHA, 2020; Mitchell et al., 1972). Respiratory acidosis is described in Section 3.2, and metabolic acidosis in Section 5.1.

4.4 VENTRICULAR ASSIST DEVICES

Patients recovering from a myocardial infarction or who are suffering from heart failure may have devices implanted to take up some or all functions of a ventricle. Patients may have a left or right ventricular assist device (LVAD or RVAD), respectively, to allow the ventricle to heal (in the case of an infarction), as a bridge to transplant, or as a permanent assist. Patients with these devices may not have palpable pulses, which makes it challenging to determine if CPR is necessary should the patient's device fails or their condition worsens. The AHA recommends that CPR be initiated if an LVAD/RVAD patient presents with abnormal skin signs with slow or non-existent capillary refill when the patient's $ETCO_2$ is less than 20 mmHg (Peberdy et al., 2017).

4.5 CARDIOGENIC OSCILLATIONS

The heart beating against the lungs can cause a small amount of gas output after normal exhalation has completed or during periods of apnea (Marks & Sidi, 2000; Smallhout & Kalenda, 1981). This will appear on the capnogram as a rippled inspiratory

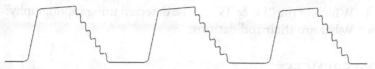

Figure 4.1 Cardiac oscillations.

downstroke, as shown in Figure 4.1, or as a rippled inspiratory baseline in apneic patients. Causes of cardiac oscillations include

- Negative intrathoracic pressure
- Pulse/respiratory ratio of at least 5.4:1 in adults and 4.0:1 in children
- Low vital capacity or heart size
- Low inspiratory–expiratory ratio
- Prolonged expiratory time
- Bradypnea or apnea
- Very low tidal volume
- Muscle relaxation (Smallhout & Kalenda, 1981)

The oscillations may result in a lower-than-actual $ETCO_2$ measurement, as some of the CO_2 is trapped in the lungs and is pulsed after passive exhalation. This may lead to the provider changing their patient treatment unnecessarily. One case report suggests that applying a small amount (5 cm H_2O) of positive end-expiratory pressure (PEEP) may relieve the oscillations (Marks & Sidi, 2000).

4.6 STUDY QUESTIONS

1 How does capnography support high-performance and pit crew resuscitation teams?

2 What is the target $ETCO_2$ range in CPR? What does it mean if the measured $ETCO_2$ is outside of this range?

3 How can capnography help us recognize return of spontaneous circulation? What do these changes indicate?

4 Which of the "Hs & Ts" can be detected using capnography? What are their indications?

REFERENCES

AHA. (2020). *Advanced Cardiovascular Life Support*. American Heart Association.

Carlson, J. N., Colella, M. R., Daya, M. R., de Maio, V. J., Nawrocki, P., Nikolla, D. A., & Bosson, N. (2021). *Prehospital cardiac arrest airway management: An NAEMSP position statement and resource document*. https://doi.org/10.1080/10903127.2021.1971349

Chicote, B., Aramendi, E., Irusta, U., Owens, P., Daya, M., & Idris, A. (2019). Value of capnography to predict defibrillation success in out-of-hospital cardiac arrest. *Resuscitation, 138*, 74–81. https://doi.org/10.1016/j.resuscitation.2019.02.028

Cone, D. C., Cahill, J. C., & Wayne, M. A. (2011). Cardiopulmonary resuscitation. In J. S. Gravenstein, M. B. Jaffe, N. Gravenstein, & D. A. Paulus (Eds.), *Capnography* (2nd ed.). Cambridge University Press.

Darocha, T., Debaty, G., Ageron, F. X., Podsiadło, P., Hutin, A., Hymczak, H., Blancher, M., Kosiński, S., Mendrala, K., Carron, P. N., Lamhaut, L., Bouzat, P., & Pasquier, M. (2022). Hypothermia is associated with a low $ETCO_2$ and low pH-stat $PaCO_2$ in refractory cardiac arrest. *Resuscitation, 174*, 83–90. https://doi.org/10.1016/J.RESUSCITATION.2022.01.022

Kodali, B. S., & Urman, R. D. (2014). Capnography during cardiopulmonary resuscitation: Current evidence and future directions. *Journal of Emergencies, Trauma, and Shock, 7*(4), 332. https://doi.org/10.4103/0974-2700.142778

Marks, R., & Sidi, A. (2000). Elimination of cardiogenic oscillations in the capnograph by applying low positive end-expiratory pressure (PEEP). *Journal of Clinical Monitoring and Computing, 16*, 177–181.

Meaney, P. A., Bobrow, B. J., Mancini, M. E., Christenson, J., De Caen, A. R., Bhanji, F., Abella, B. S., Kleinman, M. E., Edelson, D. P., Berg, R. A., Aufderheide, T. P., Menon, V., & Leary, M. (2013). Cardiopulmonary resuscitation quality: Improving cardiac resuscitation outcomes both inside and outside the hospital: A consensus statement from the American heart association. *Circulation, 128*(4), 417–435. https://doi.org/10.1161/CIR.0b013e31829d8654

Mitchell, J. H., Wildenthal, K., & Johnson, R. L. (1972). The effects of acid-base disturbances on cardiovascular and pulmonary function. *Kidney International*, *1*(5), 375–389. https://doi.org/10.1038/ki.1972.48

Peberdy, M. A., Gluck, J. A., Ornato, J. P., Bermudez, C. A., Griffin, R. E., Kasirajan, V., Kerber, R. E., Lewis, E. F., Link, M. S., Miller, C., Teuteberg, J. J., Thiagarajan, R., Weiss, R. M., & O'Neil, B. (2017). Cardiopulmonary resuscitation in adults and children with mechanical circulatory support: A scientific statement from the American Heart Association. *Circulation*, *135*(24), e1115–e1134. https://doi.org/10.1161/CIR.0000000000000504

Savastano, S., Baldi, E., Raimondi, M., Palo, A., Belliato, M., Cacciatore, E., Corazza, V., Molinari, S., Canevari, F., Danza, A. I., De Ferrari, G. M., Iotti, G. A., & Visconti, L. O. (2017). End-tidal carbon dioxide and defibrillation success in out-of-hospital cardiac arrest. *Resuscitation*, *121*, 71–75. https://doi.org/10.1016/J.RESUSCITATION.2017.09.010

Smallhout, B., & Kalenda, Z. (1981). *An Atlas of Capnography* (Revised Second). Kerckebosch-Zeist.

Touma, O., & Davies, M. (2013). The prognostic value of end tidal carbon dioxide during cardiac arrest: A systematic review. *Resuscitation*, *84*(11), 1470–1479. https://doi.org/10.1016/J.RESUSCITATION.2013.07.011

NOTES

MEDICAL EMERGENCIES

This chapter describes how capnography can be used to diagnose and manage patients with various types of medical emergencies.

5.1 METABOLIC ACIDOSIS

Acidosis can result from disturbances in the body's metabolic process. Common causes for metabolic acidosis include (Kamel & Halperin, 2017):

- *Renal failure,* resulting in excess excretion of bicarbonate, which the body needs to transport H^+ and buffered metabolic acids to the lungs.
- *Various drugs* (both licit and illicit) cause acidosis as side effects or in overdose.
- *Diabetic ketoacidosis (DKA)* leads to a build-up of acidic ketones as the body uses fat instead of glucose to generate energy.
- *Alcohol withdrawal* leads to a build-up of lactic acid due to seizures, liver insufficiency, and/or thiamine deficiency.
- *Shock states,* in particular cardiogenic shock and sepsis, lead to lactic acid build-up in the bloodstream due to anaerobic metabolism from inadequate tissue perfusion.

DOI: 10.1201/9781003491576-5

$ETCO_2$ measurements of less than 25 mmHg, with appropriate patient history, signs, and symptoms, are definitive for metabolic acidosis (Kartal et al., 2011). The low measurement indicates that

- There is insufficient bicarbonate available to remove H^+ from the hemoglobin at the lungs to be excreted as CO_2 due to metabolic acids being buffered by tissue bicarbonate (Schlichtig & Bowles, 1994; Ward, 2011).
- CO_2 production in the tissues is reduced from lack of oxygenation at the cellular level (Kamel & Halperin, 2017).

In the early stages of metabolic acidosis, patients may hyperventilate (i.e., exhibit rapid, shallow ventilation) (Kamel & Halperin, 2017). This results from an increase in CO_2 in the respiratory center due to reduced blood flow because of the acidemia; see the discussion of cerebral blood flow in traumatic brain injury in Section 7.2 and Kamel and Halperin (2017). Patients in severe metabolic acidosis may exhibit Kussmaul respirations, a deep, rapid, and labored pattern (Kamel & Halperin, 2017; Moraes & Surani, 2019). This is an ominous sign for impending respiratory failure and arrest (Moraes & Surani, 2019).

5.2 METABOLIC ALKALOSIS

Alkalosis can result from excessive loss of hydrogen ions. This can result from protracted vomiting or renal failure amongst other causes (Kamel & Halperin, 2017). Patients may present with hypoventilation and normal to high (in excess of 45 mmHg) $ETCO_2$ measurements as the body attempts to compensate for the metabolic alkalosis by retaining CO_2 (Boysen & Isenberg, 2011).

5.3 OVERDOSES: GENERAL

Drug/medication overdoses can lead to ventilatory and metabolic disturbances that need to be addressed quickly to save the patient's life. Respiratory acidosis can result from medication/drug side effects and overdoses that suppress ventilations. See the discussion on central nervous system depressant overdoses in Section 5.5.

Respiratory alkalosis can result from medication/drug side effects and overdoses by inducing hyperventilation (Boysen & Isenberg, 2011; Kamel & Halperin, 2017). Common medication/drugs that can induce hyperventilation include:

- *Salicylates*: Aspirin, bismuth subsalicylate (e.g., Pepto Bismol™), methyl salicylate (oil of wintergreen)
- *Xanthines*: Theophylline, caffeine
- *Catecholamines*: Epinephrine, norepinephrine, dopamine
- *Vasopressors*: Catecholamines, phenylephrine, vasopressin
- *Nicotine*

See the discussion on respiratory alkalosis in Section 3.3.

Drug overdoses can lead to metabolic acidosis. For example, diuretics (e.g., bumetanide, furosemide, spironolactone, hydrochlorothiazide) can cause the kidneys to excrete too much bicarbonate, leaving the body unable to buffer acids, including CO_2. See the discussion on metabolic acidosis in Section 5.1.

Drug overdoses may lead to copious and/or intractable vomiting, leading to metabolic alkalosis. Emetics given to induce vomiting (e.g., ipecac) to counteract a drug overdose or poisoning can have the same result as can the exposure to common chemicals (e.g., organophosphates). See the discussion on metabolic alkalosis in Section 5.2.

5.4 STIMULANT OVERDOSES

Stimulant overdose, in particular phencyclidine (PCP), meth-amphetamine, and 3,4-Methylenedioxymethamphetamine (MDMA, also known as Ecstasy or Molly), can lead to a hyperexcited state with delirium, decreased pain sense, increased strength, and malignant hyperthermia. When the patient can be safely evaluated, capnography can help providers to evaluate the patient's ventilatory and metabolic systems to optimize treatment. $ETCO_2$ measurements above 50 mmHg can occur, indicating

- Respiratory acidosis as the patient cannot breathe fast enough to remove the excess CO_2 being generated due to the body's hyperactivity (even if the patient has a ventilatory rate greater than 25 breaths per minute) (see Section 3.2).
- Impending malignant hyperthermia (see Section 5.6).

If the patient can breathe on their own, monitor their $ETCO_2$ measurements to ensure that they are gradually decreasing. If the patient cannot breathe on their own (e.g., due to sedative administration or the need for rapid sequence intubation), ventilate the patient at 20 breaths per minute (i.e., the high end of the range recommended in Section 3.1) until the patient's $ETCO_2$ measurements return to a normal range. Care should be taken to ensure not to hyperventilate the patient into either gastric distention and/or respiratory alka-losis. If the patient's $ETCO_2$ continues to rise, consider impending malignant hyperthermia; see Section 5.6.

5.5 CENTRAL NERVOUS SYSTEM DEPRESSANT OVERDOSES

Central nervous system depressant overdoses can lead to pro-found bradypnea and respiratory arrest, with opiate overdoses being the most common of these. In addition to hypoxia

(SpO$_2$ less than 90%), these patients may be acidotic (ETCO$_2$ greater than 45 mmHg) due to respiratory depression (see Section 3.2). Hypoxia may lead to the patient being combative upon awaking, with hypercarbia adding confusion to the mix (Kamel & Halperin, 2017). The patient should be artificially ventilated as described in Section 3.1 before administration of reversal agents to improve safety of both patient and provider (i.e., to prevent combativeness secondary to hypoxia). The patient should be artificially ventilated as described in Section 3.1 if reversal agents fail to provide adequate respiratory effort.

5.6 MALIGNANT HYPERTHERMIA

Malignant hyperthermia is a life-threatening rise in body temperature caused by muscular hypermetabolism. It may result from stimulant overdoses (see Section 5.4), paralytics used in rapid sequence intubation (e.g., succinylcholine), or anesthetic agents. Steadily rising ETCO$_2$ measurements above 50 mmHg are often the first indicator, potentially several minutes before temperature rise, of the onset of malignant hyperthermia. Malignant hyperthermia should be considered and lifesaving measures initiated if equipment failure and etiologies of CO$_2$ retention are excluded (Baudendistel et al., 1984; Gupta & Hopkins, 2017; Peng et al., 2011).

5.7 DIABETIC KETOACIDOSIS

Diabetic ketoacidosis is the result of being in a prolonged (hours to days) hyperglycemic state (blood glucose at or above 300 mg/dL). ETCO$_2$ measurements below 25 mmHg demonstrate the presence of metabolic acidosis (see Section 5.1). Thus, the combination of high blood glucose, tachypnea, and low ETCO$_2$ measurements gives the provider high confidence in a working diagnosis of diabetic ketoacidosis (Boysen & Isenberg, 2011; Chebl et al., 2016; Kamel & Halperin, 2017; Soleimanpour et al., 2013).

5.8 HIGH-ALTITUDE ILLNESSES

High-altitude illnesses occur when people acclimated to low altitudes make a relatively rapid ascent to high altitudes. This can occur at altitudes as low as 8000 ft (2500 m) but is more likely to occur at altitudes above 10,000 ft (3050 m). Symptoms may begin within 6–12 hours of ascent (Hackett & Roach, 2001). Capnography can help differentiate high-altitude-related illnesses from other conditions, which can help the provider provide the correct treatment, and avoid unnecessary evacuation of the patient to lower altitudes (the definitive treatment for all high-altitude illnesses).

The symptoms of acute mountain sickness include headache, nausea, and fatigue. Studies suggest that a person's hypoxic drive response, specifically hyperventilation, may be protective against acute mountain sickness. Patients with $ETCO_2$ measurements between 23 and 30 mmHg are unlikely to have acute mountain sickness (Douglas & Schoene, 2010).

High-altitude pulmonary edema should be considered in patients with a dry cough and $ETCO_2$ measurements less than 23 mmHg (Douglas & Schoene, 2010; Hackett & Roach, 2001). High-altitude pulmonary edema commonly strikes on the second night at altitude, and rarely after the fourth night (Hackett & Roach, 2001). Several conditions not related to altitude can mimic high-altitude pulmonary edema, including bronchospasm, heart failure, hyperventilation syndrome, mucus plugging, and pulmonary embolism.

High-altitude cerebral edema is defined by the onset of ataxia and/or altered mental status in a patient with either acute mountain sickness or high-altitude pulmonary edema (Hackett & Roach, 2001). There are no additional capnographic indications for high-altitude cerebral edema beyond those for acute mountain sickness or high-altitude pulmonary edema.

5.9 MALAISE

Capnography can help us evaluate patients with vague complaints (e.g., "I just don't feel well") or who cause the provider an unidentifiable unease (e.g., "This patient worries me, and I don't know why"). Abnormally low $ETCO_2$ measurements might cause the provider to revisit, for example, cardiac etiologies, metabolic alkalosis, or sepsis. Abnormally high $ETCO_2$ measurements might cause the provider to revisit drug/medication overdose, metabolic acidosis, or respiratory etiologies. Capnography can help the provider formulate a differential diagnosis, if not to pinpoint a diagnosis.

5.10 SYNCOPE AND NEAR-SYNCOPE

Traditionally, orthostatic vital signs (i.e., the difference between blood pressure and pulse rate measured supine and standing) have been used in the diagnostic work-up for patients who have suffered syncopal or near-syncopal episodes where there is not a readily identifiable cause (e.g., cardiac, vasovagal response). There are several problems with this approach:

- Some patients (25% to 30%) have positive orthostatic vital signs normally, thus a positive test will have limited utility (Cohen et al., 2006).
- The results, positive or negative, are not diagnostic. In other words, they do little to prune the provider's differential diagnosis (Schaffer et al., 2018).
- In the EMS and Emergency Department environments, this test is potentially unsafe for patients and providers. If the patient stands up and becomes suddenly unconscious or too weak to stand, the resulting collapse can lead to the patient or providers being unnecessarily injured.

Capnography provides a safer and more useful diagnostic approach for these patients. If the patient has sub-normal

$ETCO_2$ measurements (less than 35 mmHg), we have evidence that the patient is hypoperfused (see Chapter 6) or suffering from a metabolic disturbance (Sections 5.1 and 5.2). Measurements above 45 mmHg suggest a respiratory etiology (Chapter 3). Conversely, normal $ETCO_2$ measurements suggest that these conditions are unlikely, thus allowing the provider to focus their diagnostic efforts elsewhere. As always, the $ETCO_2$ measurements need to be viewed in the context of the patient's vital signs, history, and other diagnostic modalities (e.g., electrocardiography).

5.11 STUDY QUESTIONS

1 Why do patients with metabolic acidosis hyperventilate?

2 How can we use capnography to tell us when it is (relatively) safe to administer opioid reversal agents?

3 Why does capnography provide an earlier warning of malignant hyperthermia than body temperature?

REFERENCES

Baudendistel, L., Goudsouzian, N., Cote, C., & Strafford, M. (1984). End-tidal CO, monitoring its use in the diagnosis and management of malignant hyperthermia. *Anaesthesia, 39*, 1000–1003.

Boysen, P. G., & Isenberg, A. V. (2011). Acid-base balance and diagnosis of disorders. In J. S. Gravenstein, M. B. Jaffe, N. Gravenstein, & D. A. Paulus (Eds.), *Capnography* (2nd ed.). Cambridge University Press.

Chebl, R. B., Madden, B., Belsky, J., Harmouche, E., & Yessayan, L. (2016). *Diagnostic value of end tidal capnography in patients with hyperglycemia in the emergency department.* https://doi.org/10.1186/s12873-016-0072-7

Cohen, E., Grossman, E., Sapoznikov, B., Sulkes, J., Kagan, I., & Garty, M. (2006). Assessment of orthostatic hypotension in the emergency room. *Blood Pressure, 15*(5), 263–267. https://doi.org/10.1080/08037050600912070

Douglas, D. J., & Schoene, R. B. (2010). End-tidal partial pressure of carbon dioxide and acute mountain sickness in the first 24 hours upon ascent to Cusco, Peru (3326 meters). *Wilderness and Environmental Medicine, 21*(2), 109–113. https://doi.org/10.1016/j.wem.2010.01.003

Gupta, P. K., & Hopkins, P. M. (2017). Diagnosis and management of malignant hyperthermia. *BJA Education, 17*(7), 249–254. https://doi.org/10.1093/bjaed/mkw079

Hackett, P. H., & Roach, R. C. (2001). High-altitude illness. *New England Journal of Medicine, 345*(2), 107–114.

Kamel, K. S., & Halperin, M. L. (2017). *Fluid, Electrolyte, and Acid-Base Physiology* (5th ed.). Elsevier.

Kartal, M., Eray, O., Rinnert, S., Goksu, E., Bektas, F., & Eken, C. (2011). $ETCO_2$: A predictive tool for excluding metabolic disturbances in nonintubated patients. *American Journal of Emergency Medicine, 29*(1), 65–69. https://doi.org/10.1016/j.ajem.2009.08.001

Moraes, A. G. de, & Surani, S. (2019). Effects of diabetic ketoacidosis in the respiratory system. *World Journal of Diabetes, 10*(1), 16–22. https://doi.org/10.4239/wjd.v10.i1.16

Peng, Y. G., Paulus, D. A., & Gravenstein, J. S. (2011). Capnography during anesthesia. In J. S. Gravenstein, M. B. Jaffe, N. Gravenstein, & D. A. Paulus (Eds.), *Capnography* (2nd ed.). Cambridge University Press.

Schaffer, J. T., Keim, S. M., Hunter, B. R., Kirschner, J. M., & De Lorenzo, R. A. (2018). Do orthostatic vital signs have utility in the evaluation of syncope? *Journal of Emergency Medicine, 55*(6), 780–787. https://doi.org/10.1016/j.jemermed.2018.09.011

Schlichtig, R., & Bowles, S. A. (1994). Distinguishing between aerobic and anaerobic appearance of dissolved CO_2 in intestine during low flow. *Journal of Applied Physiology, 76*(6). https://doi.org/10.1152/jappl.1994.76.6.2443

Soleimanpour, H., Taghizadieh, A., Niafar, M., Rahmani, F., Golzari, S. E. J., & Mehdizadeh Esfanjani, R. (2013). Predictive value of capnography for suspected diabetic ketoacidosis in the emergency department. *Western Journal of Emergency Medicine, 14*(6), 590–594. https://doi.org/10.5811/westjem.2013.4.14296

Ward, K. R. (2011). The physiological basis for capnometric monitoring in shock. In J. S. Gravenstein, M. B. Jaffe, N. Gravenstein, & D. A. Paulus (Eds.), *Capnography* (2nd ed., pp. 231–238). Cambridge University Press.

NOTES

SHOCK

This chapter discusses how capnography can be used to diagnose and manage patients in various shock states.

6.1 INTRODUCTION TO SHOCK AND CAPNOGRAPHY

Shock is defined as a systemic inadequate tissue perfusion. All forms of shock are the result of decreased or impaired blood circulation. The resulting decrease in tissue perfusion causes decreased CO_2 production and increased lactic acid production resulting in metabolic acidosis (see Section 5.1). This condition reduces the amount of CO_2 returned to the lungs to be detected via capnography. Thus, in shock, a reduction in $ETCO_2$ measurements indicates worsening acidosis, not alkalosis. This allows us to confirm both the presence and degree (compensated, decompensated, or irreversible) of shock.

6.2 COMPENSATED SHOCK

In compensated shock, the body can maintain a level of perfusion that allows the body's major systems to function, albeit at a decreased level. The body induces tachycardia, tachypnea, and vasoconstriction to maintain a marginally adequate level of perfusion.

DOI: 10.1201/9781003491576-6

The provider's challenge is determining if the measured vital signs are the result of compensated shock or sympathetic nervous stimulation. For example, a patient who has been in a motor vehicle collision without obviously life-threatening injuries may present with tachycardia, tachypnea, and a normal or elevated blood pressure. The vital signs alone do not prove or disprove compensated shock.

Capnography, combined with an appropriate history and the provider's index of suspicion, can provide an indication of existing shock and an early warning of worsening shock. Since shock diminishes tissue perfusion, there will be less CO_2 being returned to the lungs. This, combined with the body's stores of bicarbonate being reduced due to increasing metabolic acidosis, will result in $ETCO_2$ measurements that are low to low-normal (28–35 mmHg) (Kheng & Rahman, 2012). These changes will be observed before more serious signs and symptoms (e.g., dropping blood pressure) develop, allowing time to take potentially lifesaving measures. Keep in mind that the drop in $ETCO_2$ indicates worsening acidosis, not alkalosis (see Section 6.1). The combination of low $ETCO_2$ measurement with tachypnea is differentiated from hyperventilation syndrome (see Section 3.4) by the history, physical examination findings, and the lack of paresthesia and (as a late sign) carpopedal spasms.

6.3 DECOMPENSATED SHOCK

When the body can no longer maintain perfusion at low-functioning levels, i.e., the body can no longer compensate for the problem, it means shock has progressed to decompensated shock. At this stage, the body's processes begin to shut down to protect the core functionality (i.e., the heart and brain). The patient's level of consciousness and blood pressure may decrease rapidly. Tachycardia and tachypnea may persist at first but will eventually fall to "normal" levels as the body attempts to preserve available oxygen reserves.

Capnography provides an earlier indication of decompensation, and the depth thereof, than other vital signs. The first warning of decompensation provided by capnography will be a drop in $ETCO_2$ measurements to 25–27 mmHg. As decompensation progresses, $ETCO_2$ measurements will continue to decrease into the low to very low range (13–25 mmHg) (Kheng & Rahman, 2012). $ETCO_2$ values that trend downward indicate decreasing systemic perfusion, with the rate of change providing an indication of the severity of the patient's condition. Keep in mind that the drop in $ETCO_2$ indicates worsening acidosis, not alkalosis (see Section 6.1).

6.4 IRREVERSIBLE SHOCK

When the body can no longer sustain even minimal functioning, irreversible shock sets in. At this point, there is no currently available medical treatment that can save the patient's life. $ETCO_2$ measurements at or below 12 mmHg indicate that resuscitation efforts are likely futile (Kheng & Rahman, 2012).

6.5 SEPTIC SHOCK

Sepsis is the result of an infection that spreads from its original source to the bloodstream. Sepsis can quickly proceed to septic shock (a form of distributive shock), which results from inflammation of the blood vessels leading to fluid loss due to leakage into the interstitial spaces. Septic shock, if not rapidly treated, can quickly lead to death. Early stages of septic shock can be identified by two or more of the following symptoms:

- Temperature greater than 38°C (100.4°F) or less than 36°C (96.8°F)
- Respiratory rate greater than 20 breaths per minute
- Heart rate greater than 90 beats per minute

These signs combined with an identifiable infection source (e.g., urinary tract infection, decubitus ulcer) and $ETCO_2$ measurements less than 25 mmHg confirm a diagnosis of septic shock (Hunter et al., 2016). See also the discussion of metabolic acidosis in Section 5.1.

6.6 HEMORRHAGIC SHOCK

Hemorrhagic shock is a sub-set of hypovolemic shock resulting from blood loss. One of the challenges in trauma care is determining whether a patient needs a transfusion before laboratory results (e.g., complete blood count) are available and, more critically, before the patient decompensates. Studies indicated that $ETCO_2$ measurements between 27 and 33 mmHg indicate (or predict) the need for blood transfusions (Day et al., 2020; Jeanmonod et al., 2019; Williams et al., 2016; Wilson et al., 2020). Note that this range straddles the region between compensated and decompensated shock; see Sections 6.3 and 6.4. The implication of this is that $ETCO_2$ measurements greater than 30 mmHg do not rule out significant trauma, as the patient may be in compensated shock (Williams et al., 2016).

6.7 CARDIOGENIC SHOCK

Cardiogenic shock is different from most forms of shock in that the amount of fluid in the "pipes" is not a part of the problem. In hypovolemic or septic shock, for example, there is insufficient fluid in the blood vessels for the heart to pump. In cardiogenic shock, there is sufficient fluid but insufficient pump capacity to move enough blood to adequately perfuse the body's systems. In some instances, cardiogenic shock responds to an increase in pre-load, i.e., an increase in the available fluid to be pumped. The problem is how to determine if a particular patient's cardiogenic shock is "fluid responsive" (Baloch et al., 2021).

One study suggests that fluid responsiveness can be determined by performing passive leg raises for 2 minutes or infusing 300 mL of a crystalloid solution, and noting the change, if any, in the patient's $ETCO_2$ measurements. An increase of 2 mmHg or more indicates that the patient's condition is "fluid responsive" (Baloch et al., 2021).

6.8 SODIUM BICARBONATE ADMINISTRATION

Administration of sodium bicarbonate ($NaHCO_3$) for metabolic and shock-induced acidosis remains controversial. Some studies indicate a reduction in acidosis, but none show an improvement in either survival to hospital discharge neurologically intact or in 28-day mortality (Coppola et al., 2021).

Attempting to increase perfusion by alkalizing the blood in these patients solves one problem but causes others. $NaHCO_3$ helps to reduce lactic alkalosis and thereby increases the hemoglobin's ability to carry O_2 to the cells, thus increasing perfusion. However, this increases CO_2 production, which may lead to respiratory acidosis if there is insufficient hemoglobin to remove the CO_2/H^+, insufficient blood circulation to the lungs, or insufficient minute volume to remove the CO_2 at the lungs. Essentially, by administering $NaHCO_3$, we trade a metabolic (lactic) acidosis for a respiratory (CO_2) acidosis. For this reason, $NaHCO_3$ was removed from the Advanced Cardiac Life Support (ACLS) cardiac arrest algorithm (Neumar et al., 2010).

Administration of $NaHCO_3$ also results in the depletion of calcium ions (Ca^{+2}) from the bloodstream. This results in reduced cardiac function, further exacerbating metabolic acidosis and shock (Coppola et al., 2021).

One study suggests that CO_2 built up from alkalization can be managed by increasing ventilation to take advantage of the available hemoglobin capacity while simultaneously administering Ca^{+2}. While the study's authors did not monitor $ETCO_2$, one would hypothesize that after administering $NaHCO_3$, the patient's $ETCO_2$ would increase. By maintaining the $ETCO_2$ in the 30–35 mmHg range, it should be possible to manage $PaCO_2$ levels. In the study, blood pH increases (i.e., becomes less acidotic) when using this strategy. What was not measured in this rat study was whether this strategy increased survival, as the rats were "sacrificed" (Kimmoun et al., 2014).

The key takeaways from this discussion are:

- The use of $NaHCO_3$ is, at best, a temporizing measure with resolution of the underlying condition being paramount.
- When $NaHCO_3$ is given, $ETCO_2$ needs to be carefully monitored and ventilation adjusted to maintain $ETCO_2$ in the 30–35 mmHg range to maintain healthy $PaCO_2$ levels.

6.9 STUDY QUESTIONS

1 What are the capnographic indicators of shock? What is the physiology behind these indications?

2 How may a provider determine whether the patient is suffering from compensated shock or hyperventilation syndrome?

REFERENCES

Baloch, K., Rehman Memon, A., Ikhlaq, U., Umair, M., Ansari, M. I., Abubaker, J., & Salahuddin, N. (2021). Assessing the utility of end-tidal carbon dioxide as a marker for fluid responsiveness in cardiogenic shock. *Cureus*, *13*(2). https://doi.org/10.7759/cureus.13164

Coppola, S., Caccioppola, A., Froio, S., & Chiumello, D. (2021). Sodium bicarbonate in different critically ill conditions: From physiology to clinical practice. *Anesthesiology*, *134*(5), 774–783. https://doi.org/10.1097/ALN.0000000000003733

Day, D. L., Terada, K. E. F., Vondrus, P., Watabayashi, R., Severino, R., Inn, H., & Ng, K. (2020). Correlation of nasal cannula end-tidal carbon dioxide concentration with need for critical resources for blunt trauma patients triaged to lower-tier trauma activation. *Journal of Trauma Nursing, 27*(2). https://doi.org/10.1097/JTN.0000000000000492

Hunter, C. L., Silvestri, S., Ralls, G., Stone, A., Walker, A., & Papa, L. (2016). A prehospital screening tool utilizing end-tidal carbon dioxide predicts sepsis and severe sepsis. *American Journal of Emergency Medicine, 34*(5), 813–819. https://doi.org/10.1016/j.ajem.2016.01.017

Jeanmonod, R., Tran, J., Thiyagarajan, D., Wilson, B., Black, J., Agarwala, S., & Jeanmonod, D. (2019). End-tidal carbon dioxide on emergency department arrival predicts trauma patient need for transfusion, vasopressors, and operative hemorrhage control in the first 24 hours. *International Journal of Academic Medicine, 5*(1). https://doi.org/10.4103/IJAM.IJAM_43_18

Kheng, C. P., & Rahman, N. H. (2012). The use of end-tidal carbon dioxide monitoring in patients with hypotension in the emergency department. *International Journal of Emergency Medicine, 5*(1). https://doi.org/10.1186/1865-1380-5-31

Kimmoun, A., Ducrocq, N., Sennoun, N., Issa, K., Strub, C., Escanyé, J. M., Leclerc, S., & Levy, B. (2014). Efficient extra- and intracellular alkalinization improves cardiovascular functions in severe lactic acidosis induced by hemorrhagic shock. *Anesthesiology, 120*(4), 926–934. https://doi.org/10.1097/ALN.0000000000000077

Neumar, R. W., Otto, C. W., Link, M. S., Kronick, S. L., Shuster, M., Callaway, C. W., Kudenchuk, P. J., Ornato, J. P., McNally, B., Silvers, S. M., Passman, R. S., White, R. D., Hess, E. P., Tang, W., Davis, D., Sinz, E., & Morrison, L. J. (2010). Part 8: Adult Advanced Cardiovascular Life Support: 2010 American Heart Association Guidelines for Cardiopulmonary Resuscitation and Emergency Cardiovascular Care. *Circulation, 122*(SUPPL. 3). https://doi.org/10.1161/CIRCULATIONAHA.110.970988

Williams, D. J., Guirgis, F. W., Morrissey, T. K., Wilkerson, J., Wears, R. L., Kalynych, C., Kerwin, A. J., & Godwin, S. A. (2016). End-tidal carbon dioxide and occult injury in trauma patients: $ETCO_2$ does not rule out severe injury. *American Journal of Emergency Medicine, 34*(11). https://doi.org/10.1016/j.ajem.2016.08.007

Wilson, B. R., Bruno, J., Duckwitz, M., Akers, N., Jeanmonod, D., & Jeanmonod, R. (2020). Prehospital end-tidal CO_2 as an early marker for transfusion requirement in trauma patients. *American Journal of Emergency Medicine.* https://doi.org/10.1016/j.ajem.2020.08.056

NOTES

TRAUMA

This chapter describes how capnography can be used to manage patients with traumatic injuries.

7.1 MAJOR TRAUMA

Studies indicate that arterial CO_2 measurements ($PaCO_2$) may be significantly higher than $ETCO_2$ measurements in severe trauma patients. This is caused by both the decrease in venous return to the lungs and the gradual depletion of bicarbonate stores. The result is that the low $ETCO_2$ may lead a provider to hypoventilate the patient to raise the $ETCO_2$, which leads to an artificially induced respiratory acidosis. These studies also indicate that acidosis is a predictor of poor patient outcomes. While our goal is to achieve $ETCO_2$ measurements in the range of 30–35 mmHg, we must ensure that proper oxygenation and ventilation are maintained throughout the shock/trauma resuscitation efforts (Cooper et al., 2013; Doppmann et al., 2021; Frakes, 2011). See Section 3.1 for recommendations for managing ventilations.

The recommended $ETCO_2$ range (30–35 mmHg) is based on two factors. First, this range is appropriate for head-injured patients, and many of our trauma patients also have traumatic brain injuries (see Section 7.2). Second, as $PaCO_2$ may be

DOI: 10.1201/9781003491576-7

significantly higher than $ETCO_2$, maintaining the patient in the recommended range keeps the patient within a normal to high range, thus minimizing or preventing respiratory acidosis.

7.2 TRAUMATIC BRAIN INJURY

Traumatic brain injury patients suffer from two related and competing problems. The injury results in cerebral swelling and edema, which reduces cerebral blood flow. Hyperventilation ($ETCO_2$ measurements below 30 mmHg) will reduce the swelling but will also reduce cerebral blood flow. Hypoventilation ($ETCO_2$ measurements above 40 mmHg) will increase cerebral blood flow but also increase swelling. The challenge then is to balance these two potentially lethal sequelae. Maintaining $ETCO_2$ between 30 and 35 mmHg balances the need to reduce swelling with the need to retain cerebral blood flow (Frakes, 2011).

The brain injury itself can complicate the situation. Bradypnea, as part of Cushing's Triad, can lead to respiratory acidosis. These patients may require artificial ventilations to support adequate $ETCO_2$ and SpO_2 values. On the other hand, the patient's injury may result in tachypnea, resulting in respiratory alkalosis. It may be necessary to paralyze and mechanically ventilate these patients.

Another complication is that studies have demonstrated that the correlation between $ETCO_2$ and $PaCO_2$ measurements is poor in patients with traumatic brain injuries (Yang et al., 2019). $PaCO_2$ is higher, often significantly, than $ETCO_2$. The significance of this finding is that withholding ventilations to raise the $ETCO_2$ to 30 mmHg is both unnecessary ($PaCO_2$ is near normal) and dangerous for the patient because oxygenation is not being maintained. Similarly, allowing $ETCO_2$ measurements greater than 35 mmHg means the patient's $PaCO_2$ is in a very unhealthy range (well above normal). These patients should be ventilated at a rate at the high end of normal; see Section 3.1.

Another way to use capnography to support the head injured patient is to combine $ETCO_2$ trend with mean arterial pressure (MAP) trend. If both MAP and $ETCO_2$ are trending downward, the patient is losing critical perfusion and needs fluid support to maintain sufficient pressure to prevent cerebral ischemia (Grayson, 2016).

7.3 BURNS

As with trauma and head injured patients, the correspondence between $ETCO_2$ and $PaCO_2$ in burn patients is poor (Cooper et al., 2013). The goal of ventilation, just as with trauma and traumatic brain injury, is to ensure adequate oxygenation ($SpO_2 \geq 94\%$), not simply to maintain $ETCO_2$ within the textbook range (see Section 3.1).

7.4 PAIN MANAGEMENT

It is tempting to use capnography, along with cardiac monitoring, to judge the degree of a patient's pain. A patient in pain may be expected to be tachycardic and to have hypercarbia due to increased metabolism from both the pain itself and the precipitating insult. The patient may also be tachypneic from either (or both) pain caused by ventilations or from CO_2 build-up. The problem with this approach is many medical problems cause tachycardia, hypercarbia, and tachypnea, thus confounding any findings. Tachycardia and abnormal capnography must be assumed to be related to the patient's medical condition and not the patient's degree of pain.

Similarly, a patient who is normocardic and normocapnic may still be experiencing considerable pain. Isolated extremity injuries can be quite painful, but the degree of sympathetic nervous system stimulation will vary between individuals.

Thus, capnography cannot be used to objectively determine a patient's level of pain.

However, capnography plays a crucial role in managing the use of pain medications that can cause central nervous system depression (e.g., narcotics, benzodiazepines), respiratory depression, and/or respiratory arrest. As noted in Section 3.13, capnography can detect and alarm respiratory changes much faster than human observation or pulse oximetry. By observing trends in the $ETCO_2$ measurements and ventilation rate, supplemented by low ventilation alarms, the provider can obtain early warning of medication-induced hypoventilation or apnea. This gives the provider time to adjust, or reverse, the medication prior to the patient becoming apneic (Burton et al., 2006; Hatlestad, 2005; Hutchison, 2006; Krauss & Hess, 2007).

Capnography can be used to help patients manage their pain when medication is contraindicated or ineffective through biofeedback. This must be explained to the patients that they need to either (or both) reduce their ventilatory rate or increase their $ETCO_2$ measurement. In many cases, the patients are able to adjust their ventilations, which improves their status (Meckley, 2009; Meuret, 2011). At the very least, this may distract the patient from their discomfort, which may improve their ventilatory status.

7.5 STUDY QUESTIONS

1 The correspondence between $ETCO_2$ and $PaCO_2$ is poor in patients with head trauma or burns. What does this imply when interpreting $ETCO_2$ measurements? How does this impact our management of these patients?

2 What role does capnography play in pain management?

REFERENCES

Burton, J. H., Harrah, J. D., Germann, C. A., & Dillon, D. C. (2006). Does end-tidal carbon dioxide monitoring detect respiratory events prior to current sedation monitoring practices? *Academic Emergency Medicine*, *13*(5), 500–504. https://doi.org/10.1197/J.AEM.2005.12.017

Cooper, C. J., Kraatz, J. J., Kubiak, D. S., Kessel, J. W., & Barnes, S. L. (2013). Utility of prehospital quantitative end tidal CO_2? *Prehospital and Disaster Medicine, 28*(2), 87–93. https://doi.org/10.1017/S1049023X12001768

Doppmann, P., Meuli, L., Sollid, S. J. M., Filipovic, M., Knapp, J., Exadaktylos, A., Albrecht, R., & Pietsch, U. (2021). End-tidal to arterial carbon dioxide gradient is associated with increased mortality in patients with traumatic brain injury: A retrospective observational study. *Scientific Reports, 11*(1), 1–9. https://doi.org/10.1038/s41598-021-89913-x

Frakes, M. A. (2011). Capnography during transport of patients (inter/intra-hospital). In J. S. Gravenstein, M. B. Jaffe, N. Gravenstein, & D. A. Paulus (Eds.), *Capnography* (2nd ed.). Cambridge University Press.

Grayson, K. (2016). *Capnography in the patient with severe neurological injury.* EMS1. https://www.ems1.com/ems-products/capnography/articles/capnography-in-the-patient-with-severe-neurological-injury-5ksMR7FvD9Fgp9b3/

Hatlestad, D. (2005). Capnography in sedation and pain management. *Emergency Medical Services, 34*(3), 65–69.

Hutchison, R. (2006). Capnography monitoring during opioid PCA administration. *Journal of Opioid Management, 2*(4), 207–208. https://doi.org/10.5055/jom.2006.0032

Krauss, B., & Hess, D. R. (2007). Capnography for procedural sedation and analgesia in the emergency department. *Annals of Emergency Medicine, 50*(2), 172–181. https://doi.org/10.1016/j.annemergmed.2006.10.016

Meckley, A. (2009). *Balancing Unbalanced Breathing: The Clinical Use of Capnographic Biofeedback. 41*(4), 183–187. https://doi.org/10.5298/1081-5937-41.4.02

Meuret, A. E. (2011). Biofeedback. In J. S. Gravenstein, M. B. Jaffee, N. Gravenstein, & D. A. Paulus (Eds.), *Capnography* (2nd ed.). Cambridge University Press.

Yang, J. T., Erickson, S. L., Killien, E. Y., Mills, B., Lele, A. V., & Vavilala, M. S. (2019). Agreement between arterial carbon dioxide levels with end-tidal carbon dioxide levels and associated factors in children hospitalized with traumatic brain injury. *JAMA Network Open, 2*(8), 1–12. https://doi.org/10.1001/jamanetworkopen.2019.9448

NOTES

NEUROLOGICAL EMERGENCIES

This chapter describes how capnography can be used to manage patients with various neurological emergencies.

8.1 STROKE

Assessing conscious and alert patients for strokes (i.e., cerebral vascular accident) does not require the use of capnography, as the presence and severity of a stroke can be evaluated using stroke scales such as the Cincinnati or (United States) National Institutes of Health (NIH) stroke scales. Capnography may be useful for patients who are unable to follow instructions where stroke is suspected. Stroke patients have been shown to have lower $ETCO_2$ measurements than people without cerebral vascular abnormalities (Minhas, 2018; Salinet et al., 2019). This may be the result of decreased metabolism in the affected brain region, or due to respiratory or circulatory effects from the insult. If it becomes necessary to artificially ventilate the patient, follow the guidelines discussed in Section 7.2 for traumatic brain injuries.

8.2 SEIZURES

Capnography can be used to reliably assess the pulmonary status of active and postictal grand mal seizure patients (Abramo et al., 1997; Bateman et al., 2008; Seyal et al., 2010).

DOI: 10.1201/9781003491576-8

Patients experiencing grand mal and complex partial seizures will be apneic or severely bradypneic during the seizure. Postictal, the patient will initially be hypercarbic (ETCO$_2$ greater than 45 mmHg) due to a build-up of metabolic by-products during the seizure, and bradypneic (Seyal et al., 2010). If artificial ventilation is necessary, the goal should be normocarbia while avoiding hypocarbia (ETCO$_2$ less than 35 mmHg) in seizure patients (Meuret, 2011); see Section 3.1.

Patients with partial seizures, including focal and absence seizures, can benefit from capnography monitoring. These seizures can spread resulting in bradypnea or apnea even if the seizures do not progress to generalized (i.e., grand mal) seizures (Bateman et al., 2008). Capnography monitors will alarm many seconds, up to a minute, prior to SpO$_2$ monitors if the patient becomes apneic or if the patient's ETCO$_2$ measurements exceed critical values; see Section 3.13.

8.3 STUDY QUESTIONS

1 How will a stroke patient's capnography differ from that of a patient with normal cerebral vasculature? Why?

2 Your patient tells you they are experiencing the aura that presages a seizure. How can capnography help in the monitoring of this patient? What will the capnography show when the patient becomes postictal?

REFERENCES

Abramo, T. J., Wiebe, R. A., Scott, S., Goto, C. S., & McIntire, D. D. (1997). Noninvasive capnometry monitoring for respiratory status during pediatric seizures. *Critical Care Medicine*, *25*(7), 1242–1246.

Bateman, L. M., Li, C. S., & Seyal, M. (2008). Ictal hypoxemia in localization-related epilepsy: Analysis of incidence, severity and risk factors. *Brain*, *131*(12), 3239–3245. https://doi.org/10.1093/brain/awn277

Meuret, A. E. (2011). Biofeedback. In J. S. Gravenstein, M. B. Jaffee, N. Gravenstein, & D. A. Paulus (Eds.), *Capnography* (2nd ed.). Cambridge University Press.

Minhas, J. S. (2018). Highlighting the potential value of capnography in acute stroke. *Journal of Emergency Medicine, 55*(1), 130–131. https://doi.org/10.1016/j.jemermed.2017.11.033

Salinet, A. S. M., Minhas, J. S., Panerai, R. B., Bor-Seng-Shu, E., & Robinson, T. G. (2019). Do acute stroke patients develop hypocapnia? A systematic review and meta-analysis. *Journal of the Neurological Sciences, 402*(February), 30–39. https://doi.org/10.1016/j.jns.2019.04.038

Seyal, M., Bateman, L. M., Albertson, T. E., Lin, T. C., & Li, C. S. (2010). Respiratory changes with seizures in localization-related epilepsy: Analysis of periictal hypercapnia and airflow patterns. *Epilepsia, 51*(8), 1359–1364. https://doi.org/10.1111/j.1528-1167.2009.02518.x

NOTES

9

DIFFERENTIAL DIAGNOSIS
Capnogram

Figure 9.1a–c provides a flow chart for the interpretation of the capnogram (Gravenstein, 2011; Ward & Yealy, 1998). Each end point (represented by an oval) identifies the chapter to refer to for more information. Chapter 10 should be consulted when the capnogram by itself is not diagnostic.

DOI: 10.1201/9781003491576-9

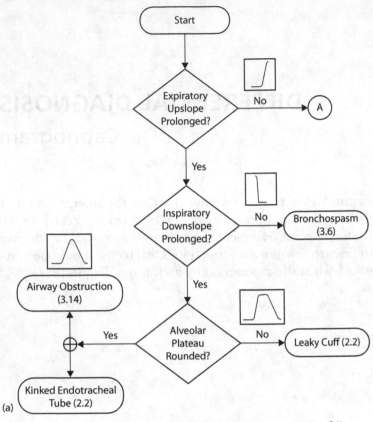

Figure 9.1 (a) Differential diagnosis based on capnogram (1 of 3).

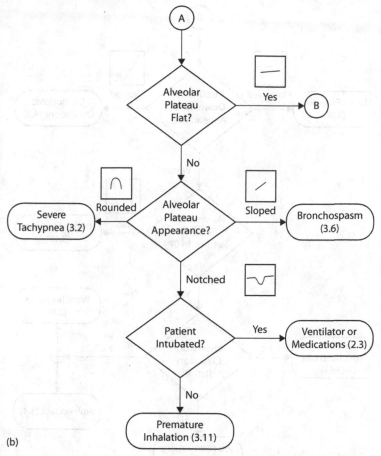

Figure 9.1 (*Continued*) (b) differential diagnosis based on capnogram (2 of 3).

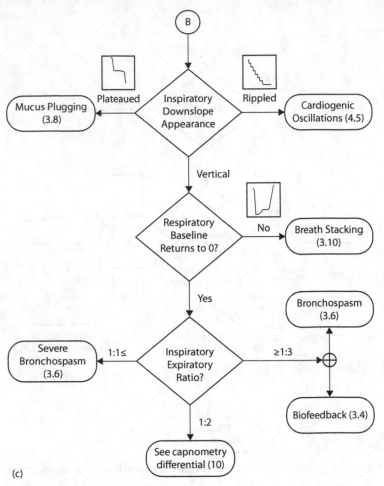

Figure 9.1 (*Continued*) (c) differential diagnosis based on capnogram (3 of 3).

REFERENCES

Gravenstein, J. S. (2011). Clinical perspectives. In D. A. Gravenstien, J. S. Jaffe, M. B. Gravenstien, N. Paulus (Eds.), *Capnography* (2nd ed.). Cambridge University Press.

Ward, K. R., & Yealy, D. M. (1998). End-tidal carbon dioxide monitoring in emergency medicine, Part 1: Basic principles. *Academic Emergency Medicine, 5*(6), 628–636. https://doi.org/10.1111/j.1553-2712.1998.tb02473.x

NOTES

10

DIFFERENTIAL DIAGNOSIS
Capnometry

Table 10.1 provides differential diagnosis suggestions for different combinations of ventilatory rate and $ETCO_2$ measurements. Each potential diagnosis includes a reference of sections for further reading elsewhere in this text.

DOI: 10.1201/9781003491576-10

Table 10.1 Differential diagnosis based on capnometry

	Bradypnea	Normopnea	Tachypnea
Hypercarbia	Metabolic alkalosis (5.2) CNS depressant overdose (5.5) Seizure (8.2)	Respiratory failure (3.12) Lower airway obstruction (3.14) Malignant hyperthermia (5.6)	Bronchospasm (3.6) Respiratory failure (3.12) Lower airway obstruction (3.14) Simulant overdose (5.4) Malignant hyperthermia (5.6)
Normocarbia	Metabolic alkalosis (5.2)	Acute mountain sickness (5.8)	V/Q mismatch (3.5) Compensated shock (6.2)
Hypocarbia	Metabolic alkalosis (5.2)	Mucus plugging (3.8) Decompensated shock (6.3) Septic shock (6.5) Hemorrhagic shock (6.6)	Hyperventilation syndrome (3.4) V/Q mismatch (3.5) Congestive heart failure (3.7) Collapsed lung (3.9) Metabolic acidosis (5.1) Diabetic ketoacidosis (5.7) High-altitude pulmonary edema (5.8) Compensated shock (6.2) Septic shock (6.5) Hemorrhagic shock (6.6)

NOTES

NOTES

CLINICAL SCENARIOS

This chapter presents several clinical scenarios to test your ability to apply capnography in real-world situations.

11.1 DIFFICULTY BREATHING

Your patient is a 60-year-old male with a chief complaint of sudden-onset, unprovoked difficulty breathing. He is tripoding, alert and oriented by four (self, place, time, and events), speaking in two- or three-word sentences, with a history of "COPD". You are unable to auscultate lung sounds. His vital signs are blood pressure 150/100, heart rate 110, SpO_2 94% at room air, ventilatory rate 28 breaths per minute and labored.

What is your differential diagnosis? How do the potential treatments differ?

You place the patient on side-stream capnography using a nasal sensor. It confirms your observed ventilatory rate, displays $ETCO_2$ measurements of 50 to 60 mmHg, and displays the capnogram shown in Figure 11.1.

DOI: 10.1201/9781003491576-11

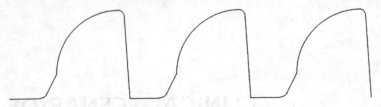

Figure 11.1 Capnogram: Scenario 1.

What do the ETCO₂ measurements indicate? What does the capnogram tell you about the cause?

You treat the patient for acute bronchospasm. His SpO_2 improves to 97% at room air, his ventilatory rate decreases to 20 breaths per minute unlabored, and the patient states that he feels "much better" (see Section 3.6).

11.2 MALAISE 1

Your patient is a 67-year-old female with a chief complaint of gradual onset over "2 days" of malaise. She complains of 3/10 suprapubic pain and states that she "recently" had a "UTI". Her medical history includes hypertension for which she takes metoprolol. The patient is afebrile, with an observed ventilatory rate of 24 breaths per minute and otherwise unremarkable vital signs.

What is your differential diagnosis? How do the treatment plans differ?

You place the patient on side-stream capnography using a nasal sensor. It confirms your observed ventilatory rate, displays ETCO₂ measurements of 18–22 mmHg, and displays the capnogram shown in Figure 11.2.

What do the ETCO₂ measurements indicate? What does the capnogram tell you about the cause? How did the patient's medication confound the diagnosis?

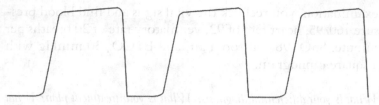

Figure 11.2 Capnogram: Scenario 2.

You initiate a "Code Sepsis" response. The patient is started on broad spectrum antibiotics and fluid resuscitation. Blood gas measurements show high serum lactate levels, confirming the diagnosis of sepsis (see Section 6.5).

11.3 SLIP AND FALL

You are called to a single-family dwelling where a party is in full swing. Your patient is a 40-year-old female sitting upright in a chair in the kitchen applying an ice pack to her forehead. Per the patient's partner, the patient has been "drinking all night", fell, and hit her head on a table. The patient is alert and oriented by two (self and events) and has an oval right temporal hematoma. The patient herself has no other complaints. The patient's initial vital signs are blood pressure 170/100, heart rate of 100, ventilatory rate of 24 breaths per minute, SpO_2 98% at room air, and $ETCO_2$ 33 mmHg with a square capnogram. You place the patient on the ambulance stretcher and move to the ambulance.

What is your differential diagnosis? What is your treatment plan? What patient care destination and transport priority are you considering?

In the back of the ambulance, you perform a head-to-toe trauma examination; the only remarkable finding is the hematoma. You obtain a 12-lead EKG, which is unremarkable. The patient's blood glucose is 160 mg/dL. As it took several minutes to get to the ambulance and perform your examination, you recheck the vital signs and find blood pressure 160/95, heart rate of 92, ventilatory rate of 20 breaths per minute, SpO_2 98% at room air, and $ETCO_2$ 30 mmHg with a square capnogram.

What is your differential diagnosis? What is your treatment plan? What patient care destination and transport priority are you considering?

You decide to bypass the local community hospital and initiate transport to the nearest trauma center. Out of an abundance of caution, you establish an intravenous access with normal saline running at "keep vein open". Halfway to the trauma center you recheck the patient's vital signs and find blood pressure 155/95, heart rate of 85, ventilatory rate of 18 breaths per minute, SpO_2 98% at room air, and $ETCO_2$ 27 mmHg with a square capnogram.

Has your treatment/transport plan changed? Why? How?

You provide an update regarding the patient's condition to the hospital, begin to run the normal saline wide-open, and ask your driver to run with lights and siren to the trauma center. On arrival, the patient is immediately taken for computer-aided tomography of her head while you provide your turnover report on the move (see Section 7.2).

11.4 MOTOR VEHICLE COLLISION 1

Your patient is a 42-year-old female who was the restrained driver in a 40-mile per hour rear-end collision. Your initial assessment determines that she is alert and oriented by four (self, place, time, and events) with mild anxiety, complaining of 2/10 lower quadrant abdominal pain, with a heart rate of 110 beats per minute, and a ventilatory rate of 28 breaths per minute. The patient denies numbness and tingling.

What is your differential diagnosis? What is your treatment plan? What patient care destination and transport priority are you considering?

In the back of the ambulance, your physical examination of the patient reveals lower quadrant abdominal tenderness with no discoloration or abrasions. You place the patient on $ETCO_2$ monitoring, which confirms your observed ventilatory rate with a square capnogram and an $ETCO_2$ measurement of 33 mmHg. The patient's blood pressure is 130/94.

What is your differential diagnosis? What is your treatment plan? What patient care destination and transport priority are you considering?

Enroute to the hospital you note an $ETCO_2$ measurement of 30 mmHg, with the patient's blood pressure being measured at 128/92, heart rate of 120, and ventilatory rate of 32 breaths per minute. You ask your driver to change your destination to the nearest trauma center and to proceed with lights and siren.

On arrival at the trauma center, the trauma surgeon performs a rapid ultrasound examination of the patient's abdomen before you move the patient to the trauma bed. She finds a moderate amount of blood in the patient's abdomen. The trauma team immediately initiates a blood transfusion while the remainder of the trauma examination takes place (see Section 6.6).

11.5 MALAISE 2

Your basic life support crew is called to the residence of a 66-year-old male, with a chief complaint of a 2-day history of increasing malaise. Your initial assessment is unremarkable with a heart rate of 75 beats per minute regular and strong, ventilatory rate of 20 breaths per minute unlabored with clear lung sounds in all fields, and an SpO_2 of 92% at room air. You place the patient on 2 l/min of oxygen via a capnography nasal cannula and move the patient to your ambulance.

What is your differential diagnosis? What is your treatment plan? What patient care destination and transport priority are you considering?

You place the patient on $ETCO_2$ monitoring, which confirms your ventilatory observation, with a square capnogram and an $ETCO_2$ measurement of 28 mmHg. The patient denies recent illness or injury and his temperature is 98.3°F orally. You arrange an intercept with an advanced life support provider and set up a 12-lead EKG.

What is your differential diagnosis? What is your treatment plan? What patient care destination and transport priority are you considering?

The paramedic obtains the 12-lead EKG, which shows a sinus rhythm with a prolonged QT interval. At her request, you initiate transport to the nearest cardiac center (see Section 6.7).

11.6 HIGH-ALTITUDE RESORT

You are working in a community hospital at a high-altitude resort. Your patient is a 27-year-old female, with a chief complaint of a gradual onset 6/10 unprovoked non-radiating "sharp" headache. Her vital signs are unremarkable, and she is Cincinnati Stroke Scale negative. She arrived at the resort earlier in day, and denies recent illness or injury, pertinent medical history, medications, and allergies.

What is your differential diagnosis? What is your treatment plan?

You place the patient on $ETCO_2$ monitoring, which shows a ventilatory rate of 18 breaths per minute, square capnogram, and a $ETCO_2$ measurement of 27 mmHg.

What is your differential diagnosis? What is your treatment plan?

A detailed work-up results in a diagnosis of a sinus infection. The patient is given appropriate medications and is discharged to enjoy the remainder of her stay.

What would be your differential diagnosis if the patient's ETCO$_2$ measurement was 37 mmHg? What treatment options might you have considered?

See Section 5.8.

11.7 MOTOR VEHICLE COLLISION 2

Your patient is a 16-year-old male who was the restrained driver in a 40-mile per hour rear-end collision. Your initial assessment determines that he is alert and oriented by four (self, place, time, and events) with mild anxiety, complaining of 2/10 paresthesia in his hands, with a heart rate of 110 beats per minute and a ventilatory rate of 28 breaths per minute.

What is your differential diagnosis? What is your treatment plan? What patient care destination and transport priority are you considering?

In the back of the ambulance, your physical examination of the patient reveals no injuries. You place the patient on ETCO$_2$ monitoring, which confirms your observed ventilatory rate with a square capnogram and an ETCO$_2$ measurement of 33 mmHg. The patient's blood pressure is 130/94.

What is your differential diagnosis? What is your treatment plan? What patient care destination and transport priority are you considering?

Enroute to the hospital you note an ETCO$_2$ measurement of 30 mmHg, with the patient's blood pressure being measured at 128/92. You initiate calming measures, including capnography-based biofeedback.

On arrival at the hospital, you note that the patient's ETCO$_2$ measurement has increased to 32 mmHg and the patient's paresthesia has resolved. You learn later that the patient was discharged with a prescription for an anxiolytic (see Section 3.4).

11.8 DIABETIC MALAISE

Your patient is a 17-year-old male presenting with a chief complaint of a 3-day history of "not feeling well". He is sitting upright in a chair in the school nurse's office. He is alert and oriented by four (self, place, time, and events), but answers questions lethargically. His friend tells you that your patient has "not been acting right" today. The patient finally tells you that he is type I diabetic but is evasive when you ask about his insulin dosing.

What is your differential diagnosis? What additional history and diagnostics do you need/want?

You measure the patient's blood glucose at 550 mg/dL. His pulse is 105 beats per minute, SpO$_2$ is 90% at room air, respirations are 28 and deep, his blood pressure is 110/85, and he has an oral temperature of 98.0°F.

What is your differential diagnosis? What is your treatment plan? What patient care destination and transport priority are you considering?

You place the patient on side-stream capnography with a nasal sensor while your partner obtains vascular access. The ETCO$_2$ monitor confirms your ventilatory observation, with a square capnogram and an ETCO$_2$ measurement of 26 mmHg. You place the patient on 10 l/min of oxygen via non-rebreather mask and ask your driver to run with lights and siren to the nearest hospital with a pediatric intensive care unit. Your partner notifies the hospital that you are bringing them a patient with diabetic ketoacidosis.

The emergency department gives you a bed assignment immediately upon your arrival. The assigned nurse and the attending physician meet you as you finish moving the patient to his bed. After your report, the nurse confirms your blood glucose measurement, and the doctor is entering treatment orders as you leave the bedside (see Section 5.7).

NOTES

STUDY QUESTION ANSWERS

12.1 CHAPTER 1

1 *What is ventilation? What is respiration? How are these represented on a capnography display?*

Ventilation refers to the movement of gases into and out of the lungs. Respiration is the exchange of gases between the blood and the cells, which occurs in capillaries. Ventilation is represented by the numeric (misnamed) respiratory rate display and by the morphology of the capnogram. Respiration is represented by the $ETCO_2$ numeric display and the peak of the alveolar plateau of the capnogram.

2 *How does CO_2 output relate to ventilation, perfusion, and metabolism?*

Ventilation is a cycle of the CO_2 measurement moving from zero to a peak and back. As perfusion decreases, the amount of CO_2 being created in the cells and returned to the lungs decreases, and vice versa. As metabolism changes from aerobic to anaerobic, the amount of CO_2 returned to the lungs decreases, and vice versa.

3 *What is the relationship between HCO_3^- and CO_2 output?*

The majority of CO_2 is carried to the lungs via the attachment of H^+ to hemoglobin. In capillaries around cells, CO_2 combines with H_2O in the blood to create H^+ and HCO_3^-.

DOI: 10.1201/9781003491576-12

This reaction is reversed in capillaries surrounding the alveoli, with the CO_2 passing through the alveoli to be exhaled and the H_2O traveling to the kidneys for excretion. A lack of HCO_3^- reduces the amount of H^+ that can be removed from the hemoglobin and thus the amount of CO_2 that can be exhaled.

4   *Name the segments of the capnogram. What does each represent? What does an abnormal presentation of each mean?*

The respiratory baseline represents exhalation from the anatomic dead space; i.e., parts of the respiratory system that do not take part in gas exchange such as the trachea and the mainstem bronchi; this should be zero. The expiratory upstroke represents a mix of dead space and alveolar exhalation. The alveolar plateau represents alveolar exhalation, with the end point representing the $ETCO_2$ value. The inhalation downstroke represents inhalation of gas that is nearly free of CO_2. A non-zero respiratory baseline suggests that exhalation is not finishing before inhalation begins. A curved or sharply angled expiratory upstroke indicates increased resistance during exhalation. A shortened or curved alveolar plateau indicates difficulty in evacuating the bottom of the bronchial tree. A sharply angled inhalation downstroke indicates resistance during inhalation.

12.2 CHAPTER 2

1   *How does a non-zero $ETCO_2$ measurement assure the provider that an advanced airway is correctly placed?*

Little to no CO_2 is present in the esophagus and stomach, and there is essentially none in room air. If an endotracheal tube is placed in the esophagus, or if a supraglottic airway is not properly sealed, ambient gases (i.e., room air) will be drawn into the sensor as the patient did not "inhale" so there will be no CO_2-rich exhalation.

2 *Why is the inspiratory downstroke sharply sloped with a leaky endotracheal tube balloon?*

When an endotracheal tube is leaky (i.e., not sealing the trachea), ambient gases are being entrained, which draws less gas through the tube, thus increasing the amount of time it takes for CO_2 in the tube to become zero.

3 *What vital sign may help in diagnosing a notched alveolar plateau? Why?*

A decreased or decreasing SpO_2 measurement may help diagnose a notched alveolar plateau. This may indicate that the patient's oxygen supply has been compromised resulting in the patient becoming (relatively or absolutely) hypoxic.

12.3 CHAPTER 3

1 *Why is it desirable to maintain $ETCO_2$ between 30 and 35 mmHg, versus the normal 35–45 mmHg, during artificial ventilations?*

This $ETCO_2$ range helps to maintain a balance between cerebral oxygenation and swelling. Increasing the oxygenation resulting in deceased $ETCO_2$ (i.e., hyperventilation) can result in increased cerebral swelling. Conversely, reducing the oxygenation resulting in increased $ETCO_2$ (i.e., hypoventilation) reduces cerebral swelling at the cost of cerebral hypoxia. This range also benefits trauma and burn patients whose $PaCO_2$ may be higher than their $ETCO_2$.

2 *What are the signs and symptoms of respiratory acidosis and respiratory alkalosis?*

Patients with respiratory acidosis will present with decreased minute ventilations and increased $ETCO_2$ measurements. Patients with respiratory alkalosis will present with normal to increased minute ventilations and decreased $ETCO_2$ measurements.

3   *What does a "shark fin" waveform indicate? Why? How can the waveform tell us if our treatment is effective?*

A waveform with a sloped or curved expiratory upstroke indicates bronchospasm. The curve results from the increased effort, and therefore the increased time, required for the patient to evacuate the alveolar tree. The waveform will gradually return to a more normal appearance as treatment relieves the bronchospasm.

4   *How can capnography help differentiate between congestive and obstructive etiologies of dyspnea?*

Congestive dyspnea will typically present with nearly normal waveforms and low to normal $ETCO_2$ measurements. Obstructive dyspnea will typically present with an abnormal expiratory upslope and increased $ETCO_2$ measurements.

12.4   CHAPTER 4

1   *How does capnography support high-performance and pit crew resuscitation teams?*

The provider responsible for ventilations uses capnography to ensure that artificial airways are properly placed and remain patent, and that their ventilation rate is neither too fast nor too slow. The provider providing compressions uses capnography to ensure that their rate and depth are appropriate. The provider leading the resuscitation effort uses capnography to monitor the overall effectiveness of the team's effort, to determine if shocks (particularly the first) are appropriate, if spontaneous circulation returns, and as an aid in determining if further efforts may be futile.

2   *What is the target $ETCO_2$ range in CPR? What does it mean if the measured $ETCO_2$ is outside of this range?*

The target $ETCO_2$ range is 10–20 mmHg. Measurements less than 10 mmHg may indicate too frequent ventilation or inadequate compressions. Measurements above 20 mmHg may indicate ventilations are not frequent enough or that compressions are inadequate.

3   *How can capnography help us recognize return of spontaneous circulation? What do these changes indicate?*

A sudden and sustained increase in $ETCO_2$ measurements above 20 mmHg indicates that spontaneous circulation has returned. The increased $ETCO_2$ results from improved perfusion especially in the heart and brain, and from increased cardiac and brain activity.

4   *Which of the "Hs & Ts" can be detected using capnography? What are their indications?*

Capnography can be used to detect "hydrogen ions", i.e., acidosis. In a patient with spontaneous circulation, $ETCO_2$ measurements below 25 mmHg indicate a metabolic acidosis, while measurements above 45 mmHg indicate a respiratory acidosis.

12.5 CHAPTER 5

1   *Why do patients with metabolic acidosis hyperventilate?*

Hyperventilation is a ventilatory rate in excess of biological requirements (see Section 4.4). As cerebral perfusion declines, CO_2 builds up in the areas of the brain responsible for ventilation. The normal drive for ventilation is hypercarbia. With decreased perfusion, the brain overestimates the amount of CO_2 in the system and induces increasing ventilatory rates to reduce the erroneously detected hypercarbia.

2   *How can we use capnography to tell us when it is (relatively) safe to administer opioid reversal agents?*

Patient's SpO_2 and $ETCO_2$ measurements returning to relatively normal values (at least 94% and less than 45 mmHg, respectively) indicate that the likelihood of hypoxia/ hypercarbia induced combativeness has been minimized and is therefore (relatively) safe to administer reversal agents.

3 *Why does capnography provide an earlier warning of malignant hyperthermia than body temperature?*

Heat and CO_2 are by-products of metabolism. Hypermetabolism generates excess amounts of both. The body has several mechanisms for removing heat, and these mechanisms are built to respond very quickly to temperature changes. It takes a relatively long time to overwhelm the thermoregulatory system. In contrast, the body has essentially only one way to remove excess CO_2, the respiratory system, which is relatively easy to overwhelm. Thus, the CO_2 will build up more quickly than the temperature will rise, providing an early indication of malignant hyperthermia.

12.6 CHAPTER 6

1 *What are the capnographic indicators of shock? What is the physiology behind these indications?*

A patient in shock will present with tachypnea and $ETCO_2$ measurements at or below 30 mmHg. Patients in shock are acidotic, which reduces the ability of hemoglobin to carry oxygen. The patient ventilates more rapidly in an effort to remove acid (i.e., CO_2) from the body and to bring in more oxygen. Because the body is hypoperfused in shock, the cells produce less CO_2. Since the body is acidotic, HCO_3^- availability is reduced, which reduces the body's ability to remove H^+ from the hemoglobin for excretion as CO_2.

2 *How may a provider determine whether the patient is suffering from compensated shock or hyperventilation syndrome?*

A patient with hyperventilation syndrome will often present with carpopedal spasms. These result from the patient becoming alkalotic due to the removal of too much CO_2. The provider's index of suspicion is arguably more important. If there is any doubt as to which condition the provider is seeing, treat for shock as this will kill the patient whereas hyperventilation syndrome will not.

12.7 CHAPTER 7

1 *The correspondence between $ETCO_2$ and $PaCO_2$ is poor in patients with head trauma or burns. What does this imply when interpreting $ETCO_2$ measurements? How does this impact our management of these patients?*

$PaCO_2$ is higher than $ETCO_2$ in this patient population. Thus, a patient with a low to normal $ETCO_2$ measurement is actually normocarbic, and a patient with a high $ETCO_2$ measurement is actually in an acidotic state. For the patient with a low $ETCO_2$ measurement, we must not hypoventilate the patient in an attempt to raise the $ETCO_2$ to a textbook normal range. In the case of the hypercarbic patient, we need to gradually reduce the CO_2 level while avoiding hyperventilation, which could cause an overshoot and reduce the CO_2 level to dangerous levels.

2 *What role does capnography play in pain management?*

Capnography cannot be used to gauge a patient's pain perception. It can be used to ensure that we do not overdose our patients on pain medication that can cause central nervous system depression. Capnography monitors can alert a provider to patients with decreasing ventilatory rates, thus allowing the provider to intervene much sooner than using SpO_2 monitoring alone.

12.8 CHAPTER 8

1   *How will a stroke patient's capnography differ from that of a patient with normal cerebral vasculature? Why?*

A stroke patient will present with comparatively low $ETCO_2$ measurements. This is due to reduced cerebral metabolism, and possible cardiovascular or respiratory compromise due to the cerebral insult.

2   *Your patient tells you they are experiencing the aura that presages a seizure. How can capnography help in the monitoring of this patient? What will the capnography show when the patient becomes postictal?*

The patient will become apneic or severely bradypneic once the seizure starts. This will be "caught" and alarmed by the capnography monitor earlier (minutes before) than it would be by an SpO_2 monitor. Postictal, the patient will be bradypneic and hypercarbic.

NOTES

GLOSSARY

Acidosis   A state where the body's pH is acidic (less than 7.35).

Alkalosis   A state where the body's pH is alkalotic (greater than 7.45).

Alveolar plateau   The portion of a capnogram representing alveolar exhalation.

Biofeedback   A technique that uses a monitoring device (e.g., capnography) to allow a patient to perceive and control a bodily function (e.g., ventilation).

Bradypnea   Ventilatory rate less than 10 breaths per minute

Bronchospasm   Excessive constriction of the bronchioles caused by muscular contractions.

Capnogram   A waveform (i.e., graphic) display showing the amount of exhaled CO_2 over time.

Capnography   A monitoring system that measures and displays exhaled CO_2.

Capnometry   Numeric display of ventilatory rate and CO_2 measurements calculated by a capnography device.

Carpopedal spasms   Muscular spasms in the fingers and toes resulting from respiratory alkalosis.

Cincinnati Stroke Scale   An algorithm to diagnose strokes in the prehospital environment, developed by the University of Cincinnati Medical Center.

Cushing's Triad   Widening pulse pressure, decreasing pulse rate, and decreasing ventilatory rate resulting from an intracranial bleed.

Delirium A transient disturbance in level of consciousness, which may be accompanied by delusions and hallucinations.

Differential diagnosis An ordered list of potential diagnoses, with the deadliest possibilities at the top.

Eucarbia The state of having a healthy amount of CO_2 in the bloodstream ($PaCO_2$ of 35–45 mmHg).

Expiratory upstroke The portion of a capnogram representing a mix of dead space and alveolar exhalation.

Habitus A patient's physical build.

Homeostasis Steady state balance of chemical and physical processes within an organism.

Hypercarbia Excess CO_2 which manifests as $ETCO_2$ greater than 45 mmHg.

Hypocarbia Inadequate CO_2 which manifests as $ETCO_2$ less than 35 mmHg.

Inhalation downstroke The portion of a capnogram representing inhalation of gas that is nearly free of CO_2.

Inspiratory–expiratory ratio The ratio of the amount of time spent on inspiration (i.e., inhalation) versus expiration (i.e., exhalation) during one ventilatory cycle (i.e., breath).

Malaise A feeling of being unwell without a readily identifiable cause which may accompanied by fatigue and/or unease.

Malignant hyperthermia A life-threatening rise in body temperature resulting from a hypermetabolic state.

Mean arterial pressure Average circulatory system pressure during one cardiac cycle, calculated as diastolic pressure + (1/3) * (Systolic pressure − Diastolic pressure).

Metabolism Body processes that convert oxygen and nutrients to energy and waste products.

Minute ventilation The volume of gases moved into and out of the lungs in one minute.

NIH Stroke Scale An algorithm to quantify the degree of impairment resulting from a stroke, developed by the United States National Institutes of Health.

Normocarbia Normal amount of CO_2 which manifests as $ETCO_2$ measurements between 35 and 45 mmHg.

Paresthesia "Pins-and-needles" sensation resulting from pressure or damage to peripheral nerves.

Partial pressure The pressure of a component gas (e.g., oxygen) within a mixture of gases (e.g., air).

Perfusion Circulation of blood to cells throughout the body.

Pneumonia Lung infection (viral or bacterial) resulting in fluid build-up in the lungs.

Positive end–expiratory pressure Pressure maintained in the lungs (either artificially or biologically) to prevent alveolar or bronchiole collapse at the end of expiration (i.e., exhalation).

Postictal The period after a seizure characterized by an altered mental status.

Psychosis A derangement in thought and/or emotions that causes the patient to lose the ability to discern external reality.

Pulse oximetry Electronic system that measures hemoglobin saturation by measuring the absorption of light in capillary beds.

Rapid sequence intubation The process of sedating and paralyzing a patient so they can be emergently intubated.

Respiration The exchange of gases in the capillaries.

Respiratory baseline The portion of a capnogram representing exhalation from the anatomic dead space, i.e., parts of the respiratory system that do not take part in gas exchange such as the trachea and mainstem bronchi; this should be zero.

Shock Body system dysfunctions caused by inadequate tissue perfusion.

Somnolence A state of being drowsy or sleepy.

Tachypnea Ventilatory rate greater than 20 breaths per minute.

Tripoding, tripod position A seated patient leaning forward supported by one or both arms, with their head tilted upward.

Ventilation The movement of gas into and out of the lungs.

Ventilatory status The patient's rate, depth, and effort of ventilations (i.e., breathing).

INDEX

Note: Locators in *italics* represent figures and **bold** indicate tables in the text.